LOW-CARB RECIPES 2022

100 EASY, HEALTHY

AND DELICIOUS LOW CARB RECIPES

WILFRID STEPHENSON

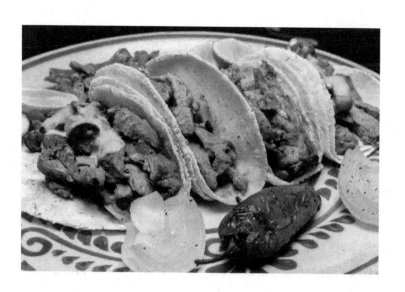

Table of Contents

INTRODUCTION

In addition to pure sugar, too many carbohydrates are responsible for unwanted weight gain with growing love handles. One reason that low carb is an ongoing trend. The low carb diet (translated: few carbohydrates) is about a drastic reduction in carbohydrates in the diet. Because only when the intake of sugar and carbohydrates is reduced does the body fall back on its energy reserves (fat pads) and thus ensure weight reduction in the event of a supposed lack of food.

So to get rid of the unpopular love handles, the diet with recipes with no or less carbohydrates is particularly effective. However, it should be noted that existing fatty tissue cells only empty themselves during the diet and then remain in the body. If you revert to your old, unhealthy eating style too quickly, you will replenish yourself quickly.

Which foods are allowed on a low carb diet?

As soon as you eat according to the low carb method, i.e. the number of carbohydrates in the food is reduced, the proportion of fat and protein that is not stored in the body to the same extent may be increased at the same time. In contrast to other forms of diet, there is no calorie deficit associated with a feeling of hunger. More fats and protein also create a longer-lasting feeling of satiety. So don't go hungry, but replace sugar and carbohydrates with high-protein, low-carbohydrate dishes.

You should avoid these foods

The following foods are the main culprits for unwanted weight gain. In addition to every form of sugar, this includes potatoes, rice and all products made from wheat flour such as pasta, pizza and bread. Their unchecked consumption becomes noticeable when consumed too high, converted into sugar, as an unpopular and often constantly growing fat reserve.

In addition, one should avoid all forms of honey and sugar, jams, Nutella, all sweets, artificial sweeteners and industrially produced juices in low carb dishes. In the case of grain and vegetables, potatoes, rice, all wheat flour products such as pizza, bread, pastries, cakes and noodles, and all industrially manufactured finished products are to be avoided. Also, a few particularly starchy foods such as bananas, corn, parsnips, sweet potatoes, peas and muesli are not necessarily recommended.

How good is low carb and how can a yo-yo effect be avoided?

If you want to avoid the dreaded yo-yo effect of rapid weight gain after the reduction diet, a general change in the eating habits that you have come to love is inevitable. The adaptation of eating behavior to age also plays an important role. In old age, unlike in younger years, the body builds up extensive fat reserves more quickly due to hormonal changes. A strict short-term switch to low carb works wonders here. However, nutritionists advise against a permanent, strict diet according to the specifications of low carb. To avoid the yo-yo effect, they recommend a balanced diet with around 50% carbohydrates afterwards. So you don't have to go without your beloved bread, potatoes and delicious pasta all the time.

LOW CARB RECIPES

1. Mojito: The Original Recipe

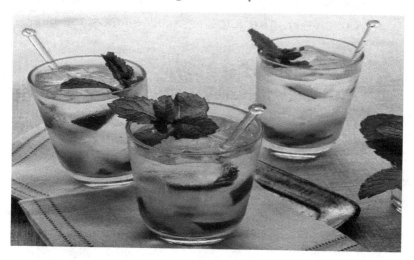

INGREDIENTS

- 20 mint leaves.
- powdered sugar.
- cuban rum
- 3 lemons green.
- sparkling water

PREPARATION

1. Crush 20 mint leaves with 5 tbsp. teaspoon of powdered sugar in a container, add 30 cl of Cuban rum, the juice of 3 large limes and mix well.
2. Pour into 6 glasses, then extend with a little sparkling water such as Perrier and a little crushed ice.
3. Decorate with mint leaves.

2. Rolled Cookie: Basic Recipe

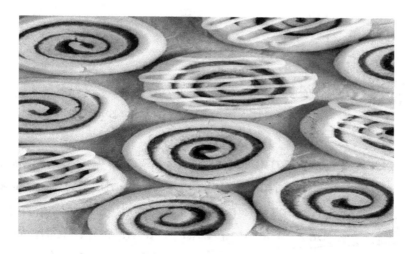

INGREDIENTS

- 120 g of sugar + 1 tsp. with coffee.
- 4 eggs
- 120 g flour.
- 25 g of melted butter

PREPARATION

1. Preheat the oven to th. 7/210 °.
2. Take the drip pan out of the oven and place a sheet of baking paper on it.
3. Separate the egg yolks from the whites, whisk the yolks and sugar until the mixture whitens and add the flour while stirring.
4. Beat the egg whites until stiff with the teaspoon of sugar, mix them gently, lift the preparation, and add the melted butter.
5. Spread the dough on the baking paper using a spatula, forming a rectangle.
6. Bake 8 minutes, take the biscuit out of the oven, place it with the baking paper on the work surface and cover it with a damp cloth.
7. Leave to stand for 10 minutes, remove the tea towel, turn the biscuit over, roll it up on itself and wrap it in film until use.

3. Low Fat Mac And Cheese

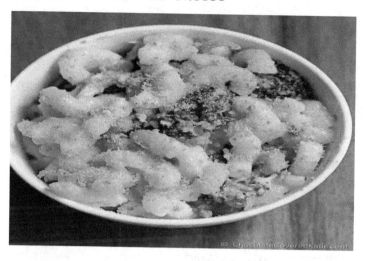

INGREDIENTS

- .1 1/2 t. of macaroni cooked and drained.
- 1 small onion, chopped.
- 9 slices, 2/3 oz strong low fat cheddar cheese.
- 1 12 oz can of evaporated skim milk.
- 1/2 t. low sodium chicken broth.
- 2 1/2 tablespoon (s) tablespoon of flour of wheat around
- .1/4 teaspoon worcestershire sauce.
- 1/2 teaspoon dry mustard.
- 1/8 teaspoon (s) of pepper.
- 3 tablespoon (s) of breadcrumbs.
- 1 tablespoon (s) of margarine, softened

PREPARATION

1. A deep baking dish sprayed with vegetable oil spray, spread 1/3 of the macaroni, 1/2 of the onions and cheese. Repeat layers, ending with macaroni. Whisk milk, broth, flour, mustard, Worcestershire sauce and pepper until combined. Pour over the layers. Combine breadcrumbs and margarine, then sprinkle on top. Bake uncovered at 375 degrees for 30 minutes until hot and bubbling.

4. A Veggie Recipe

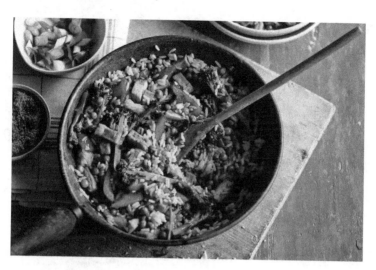

INGREDIENTS

- .2 onions.
- 2 carrots.
- 1 parsnip.
- 1 fennel
- .250 g of cereals.
- olive oil.
- turmeric salt, pepper.
- pumpkin seeds

PREPARATION

1. Brown over medium heat: sliced onions, add turmeric as desired, pepper well, then add 2 carrots (here 1 violet, 1 yellow), 1 parsnip, 1 diced fennel, salt and pepper, cook, stirring occasionally in time

2. Cook 1 250g packet of cereals in boiling salted water (like bulgur quinoa from Monoprix, which cooks in 10 minutes), drain, pour into a salad bowl, season with 2 tbsp. tablespoons olive oil, pour the vegetables on top, sprinkle with roasted squash seeds for 3 minutes in a pan.

5. Burgers With Creamy Sauce And Fried Cabbage

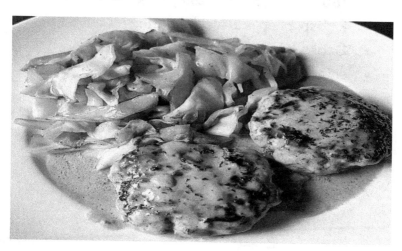

INGREDIENTS

- Burgers
- 650 g minced meat (ground)
- 1 egg
- 85 g feta cheese
- 1 tsp. Salt
- $\frac{1}{4}$ tsp. ground black pepper
- 55 g (220 ml) fresh parsley, finely chopped
- 1 tbsp. olive oil, for frying
- 2 tbsp. butter, for frying

sauce

- 180 ml cream (or cream) to whip
- 2 tbsp. chopped fresh parsley
- 2 tbsp. tomato paste or ajvar sauce
- salt and pepper

Fried green cabbage

- 550 g shredded white cabbage
- 85 g butter
- salt and pepper

Instructions

Cream burgers:

1. Mix all the ingredients for the hamburgers and assemble eight of them, longer than they are wide.
2. Fry them over medium heat in butter and olive oil for at least 10 minutes or until the patties take on a delicious color.
3. Add the tomato paste and the whipping cream to the skillet when the burgers are almost done. Mix and let the cream come to a boil.
4. Sprinkle chopped parsley on top before serving.

Green cabbage fried in butter:

1. Cut the cabbage into strips or use a food processor.
2. Melt the butter in a frying pan.
3. Sauté the shredded cabbage over medium heat for at least 15 minutes or until the cabbage is the desired color and texture.
4. Mix frequently and lower the heat a little towards the end. Season to taste.

6. Jesuit Recipe

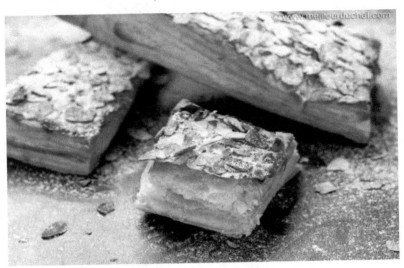

INGREDIENTS

- .50 g of almond powder.
- 50 g sugar.
- 50 g butter
- .1 egg.
- 1 liqueur glass (s) of rum

PREPARATION

1. Make two thin puff strips, 12 cm wide.
2. Garnish with a thin layer of almond cream.
3. Wet both edges with water using a brush. Place the second roll on top, press the edges to weld them.
4. Brown the surface with the egg and sow powdered almonds on top. Cut the strip thus obtained into triangles placed on a baking sheet and bake in a hot oven.
5. Sprinkle with icing sugar when you take it out of the oven. Soften the butter to cream, add the almonds and sugar at the same time.
6. Work vigorously with a whisk to obtain a frothy composition. Add the whole egg, then the Rum.

7. Chocolate Ice Cream Recipe

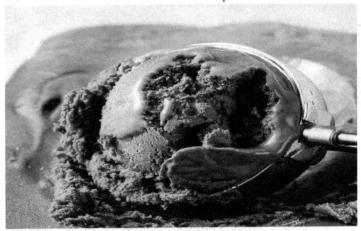

INGREDIENTS

- .6 egg yolks.
- 200 g sugar.
- 1/2 l of milk
- .300 ml of liquid sour cream.
- 100 g unsweetened cocoa

PREPARATION

1. To make your chocolate ice cream recipe:
2. Boil the milk .
3. Beat the yolks and 150g of sugar until the mixture turns white.
4. Add the cocoa and mix.
5. Pour in the milk slowly, stirring to obtain a very liquid preparation. Reheat the whole over low heat so that it thickens (without boiling it).
6. Let this juice cool.
7. Beat the cream and the rest of the sugar vigorously. Incorporate the preparation into the juice. Turbine

8. Polish Perogies, Homemade Recipe

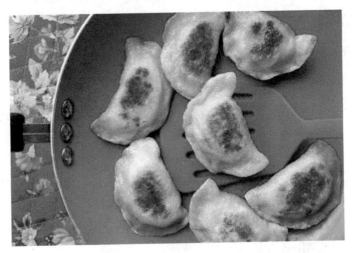

INGREDIENTS

- .2 pounds drained cottage cheese or cheese costs.
- 10 t. water.
- 1 t. lightly toasted bread crumbs.

- 3 tablespoon (s) of oil
- .4 large eggs, beaten.
- 1 1/2 teaspoon (s) of salt.
- 2 t. of flour , all purpose plus enough to prepare the dough

PREPARATION

1. In a medium bowl, mash the cheese with a fork. Incorporate the eggs, $\frac{1}{2}$ tsp. salt, flour, and mix to form a paste. Roll the dough onto a floured board and divide into 4 pieces. Spread each piece into a 12 '' long and 2 '' wide rectangle. Cut each piece diagonally to make about 10 pieces. Bring the water to a boil and add 1 tsp. desel. Reduce the heat so that the water boils slightly and immerse a third of the ravioli in it. Simmer, uncovered, until they come back up. Remove them with a skimmer, drain them. Repeat until all donuts are cooked. Serve with a little toasted bread crumbs.
2. Makes about 40 perogies.

9. Granola Basic Recipe

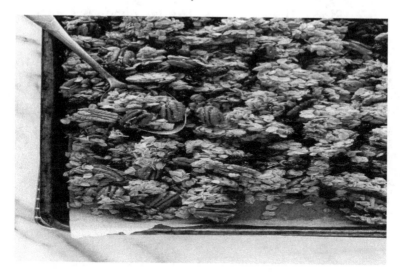

INGREDIENTS

- .300 g oatmeal.
- 100 g of whole almonds.
- 100 g of sunflower seeds.
- 100 g of pumpkin seeds.
- 50 g sesame seeds.
- 50g of grapes dry
- .10 cl of hot water.
- 50 g of liquid honey.
- 4 tablespoon (s) of cold pressed sunflower oil.
- 1 teaspoon of vanilla powder.
- 1 little sea salt

PREPARATION

1. Turn the oven on th. 5/150 °.
2. Place the oatmeal, seeds, almonds, raisins, salt and vanilla in a bowl.
3. Mix the hot water, honey and oil and pour into the bowl.
4. Stir until the liquid is absorbed, then spread the mixture on the baking sheet lined with a sheet of parchment paper.
5. Cook for 30 to 45 minutes, stirring occasionally. Let cool and set aside in a box.

10. Basic Recipe Cake

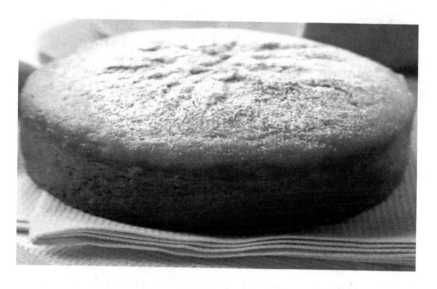

INGREDIENTS

- .100 g dark chocolate.
- 200 g of butter + 1 nut.
- 100 g of sugar + 1 little.
- 4 eggs.100 g flour
- .50 g of cornstarch.
- 30 g unsweetened cocoa.
- 1 level teaspoon of baking powder.
- 1 teaspoon of vanilla powder or cinnamon

PREPARATION

1. Turn the oven on th. 6/180 °.
2. Butter a pan and sprinkle it with a little sugar.
3. Melt the chocolate broken into pieces and the butter in the microwave or a double boiler.
4. Whisk the whole eggs and the sugar until the mixture turns white and mix them with the melted chocolate and butter.
5. Add the flour, cornstarch, cocoa, baking powder, vanilla or cinnamon. You can mix this dough using a food processor or a mixer.
6. Pour it into the mold and bake in the oven for 30 to 40 minutes. A knife point stuck in the center should come out almost dry.
7. Turn out the cake and let it cool on a wire rack.

11. Morel Mushroom Recipe

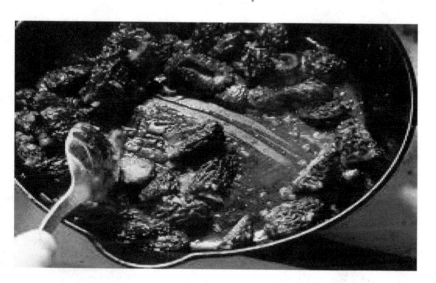

INGREDIENTS

- .250 g of morels.
- 2 veal kidneys.
- 400 g of reefing calf.
- 75 g butter.
- 5 cl of cognac
- .15 cl of sour cream.
- 4 vol au vent.
- coarse salt.
- ground pepper

PREPARATION

1. Remove the earthy part of the morels, rinse them in several waters, drain them and dry them in absorbent paper.
2. Pass the sweetbreads under a stream of cold water, blanch them for 5 minutes in salted water then drain them.
3. Open the kidneys, dice them, sauté them in 25 grams of hot butter for 8 minutes.
4. Flambé with half the cognac.
5. Cut the veal sweetbreads and brown them for 3 minutes in 25 grams of hot butter.
6. Flambé with the rest of the cognac, add half the crème fraîche, heat for 1 minute.
7. Brown the morels in the rest of the butter for 10 minutes, drain them then add the rest of the cream.
8. In a sauté pan, pour the three preparations, salt and pepper, heat for 3 minutes over low heat.
9. Place the hot preparation in the warmed crusts and serve hot.

12. French Toast: Basic Recipe

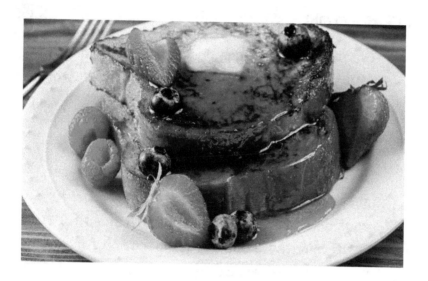

INGREDIENTS

- .50 cl of milk.
- 150 g of sugar.
- 1 vanilla pod.
- 3 eggs
- .cinnamon powder.
- 50 g butter.
- 10 slices of sandwich bread, stale baguette brioche

PREPARATION

1. Heat the milk, sugar and vanilla split in half and scraped in a saucepan and let infuse for 10 minutes, covered.
2. Beat the eggs in an omelet with 1 little cinnamon.
3. Melt half the butter in a pan, dip half of the slices of bread in the milk, then in the beaten eggs and brown in the pan on both sides for 6 to 10 minutes. Repeat the operation for the rest of the slices. Serve immediately.

13. Chocolate Cookie Recipe

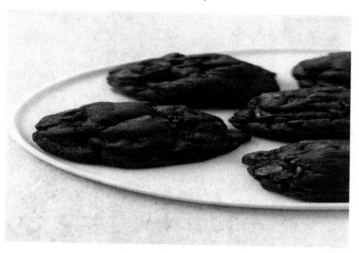

INGREDIENTS

- 200g of chocolate.
- 125g of sugar
- 125g of almond powder.
- 3 egg whites

PREPARATION

1. Preheat the oven to 180 ° C.
2. Melt the chocolate over low heat.
3. Beat the egg whites, continue beating, incorporating the sugar and ground almonds.
4. Stir in the chocolate.
5. On a baking sheet, make small piles.
6. Bake for 15 minutes.
7. Enjoy your little chocolate cookies!

14. Escalivada: The Picnic Recipe

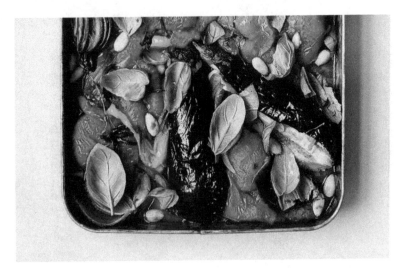

INGREDIENTS

- .2 eggplants.
- 2 zucchinis.
- 1 green pepper.
- 1 red pepper
- .6new onions.
- 2 dl of banyuls vinegar
- 2 dl olive oil.
- salt

To serve :

- .toasted bread slices
- .anchovy fillets in olive oil

PREPARATION

Turn on the oven to 210 ° C (th. 7). Rinse the eggplants, zucchini and peppers, then place them on the onions without peeling them. Slide the baking sheet into the oven. Count

1. Between 30 and 50 minutes, turning and watching the vegetables: the eggplants are cooked when they are soft under the finger's pressure, the peppers and onions when the skin is brown.

Peel

1. When lukewarm, the vegetables cut the peppers and eggplants into long strips, the onions and zucchini in half lengthwise.

Put away

1. The vegetables in a salad bowl or an airtight box. Cover them with oil and vinegar. Salt and mix gently. Serve the escalivada at room temperature or cold, accompanied by toasted slices of bread and anchovy fillets.

15. Chocolate Profiteroles - Easy Recipe

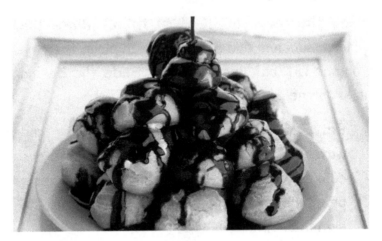

INGREDIENTS

- .for 40 small round cabbages.
- a 1.5 cm socket.

for the pastry cream:.

- custard
- .è 15 cl of whipped cream.

for the chocolate sauce :.

- 150 g dark chocolate.milk

PREPARATION

1. Gently incorporate the 15 cl of whipped cream into the pastry cream using a whisk, to lighten the cream.
2. Then, using the pastry bag, fitted with the 1.5 cm nozzle, stuff the 40 puffs, and put them in the fridge.
2. 3.Melt the chocolate in a saucepan over low heat, adding milk, until a well-bound sauce forms.
3. Arrange the cabbage in a pyramid in a dish, and cover them with lukewarm sauce.
4. Your chocolate profiteroles are ready, enjoy !
5. Discover our recipes selections: festive chocolate recipes , chocolate cake recipes, recipes of sweets ...

16. Tartiflette - Recipe From Chalet De Pierres

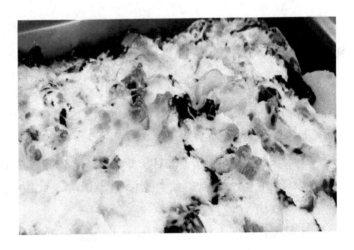

INGREDIENTS

- 1 kg of potatoes 1 onion.
- 200 g lardons 1 farmer reblochon
- 1 tablespoon (s) of crème fraîche (optional).
- 1 tablespoon (s) of vegetable oil (sunflower, peanut)
- 10 g of butter

PREPARATION

1. Cook the potatoes with their skins in a saucepan of boiling water.
2. During this time, peel and slice the onion, sweat it in hot oil, and add the bacon and brown the whole, stirring often.
3. Preheat the oven to th. 8/220 °. Butter a gratin (or cast iron) dish, pour in half the potatoes, and add half of the onion-bacon mixture, the rest of the potatoes and the rest of the onion-bacon.
4. Even out the surface, add the cream (optional) and place the whole reblochon in the center. Ground pepper and put in the oven until the top of the tartiflette is nicely browned. Serve immediately.

17. Classic Recipe Brownies

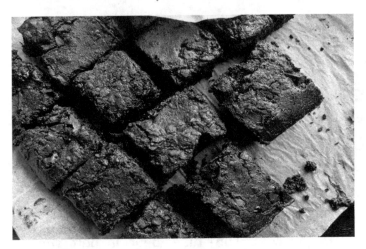

INGREDIENTS

- .125 g butter.
- 150 g of sugar.
- 4 eggs.
- 125 g chocolate
- .50 g flour.
- yeast.
- sugar ice

PREPARATION

1. Preheat your oven thermostat 6 - 7 (180 ° - 200 °).
2. Melt the butter in a saucepan over very low heat.
3. Mix the melted butter with the sugar in a bowl.
4. Add the eggs.
5. In a saucepan over very low heat, melt the chocolate cut into squares, then add it to your mixture.
6. Add the flour mixed with the salt and the baking powder.
7. Mix everything well (50 turns)
8. Put the mixture in a well buttered mold. The ideal is to use a square ceramic mold approximately 20 x 25 centimeters.
9. Put in the oven for 30 to 35 minutes. The brownie should not be overcooked.
10. Let cool, sprinkle it with icing sugar to have a more presentable white top and cut it into square pieces (for example 2 centimeters by 2 centimeters).

18. Speculoos, Simplified Recipe

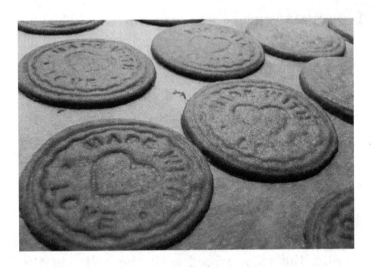

INGREDIENTS

- .250 g butter.
- 350 g flour, sifted.
- 200 g brown sugar
- .5g baking soda.

- 1 egg.
- 1 tablespoon of salt

PREPARATION

1. The preparation of speculoos requires a wait of 12 hours.
2. Mix 40g of flour, baking soda and salt in a first container.
3. Melt the butter.
4. Put it in a second container, add the brown sugar, the egg and mix vigorously. Then add the remaining flour while stirring. Mix everything and let stand 12 hours in the refrigerator.
5. After the 12 hour wait, butter baking sheets.
6. Roll out the dough, keeping a minimum thickness (3 millimeters maximum) and cut it using molds of your choice.

7. Bake everything for 20 minutes, watching the cooking.
8. It is best to let the speculoos cool before eating !

19. Scrambled Eggs With Basil And Butter

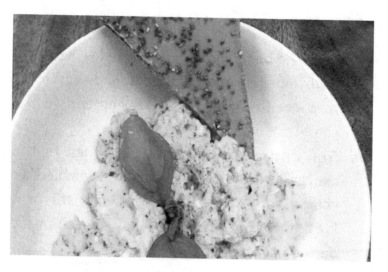

INGREDIENTS

- 2 tbsp. Butter
- 2 eggs
- 2 tbsp. cream (or cream) to mount
- salt and ground black pepper
- 80 ml (38 g) grated cheddar cheese
- 2 tbsp. fresh basil

PREPARATION

1. Melt the butter in a skillet over low heat.
2. Add the eggs, cream, cheese, and seasonings to a small bowl. Beat lightly and add to the pan.
3. Stir with a spatula from the edges to the center until the eggs have been scrambled. If you prefer them soft and creamy, stir at a low temperature until they reach your desired consistency.
4. Finish by sprinkling the basil on top.

20. Garlic Chicken Breast

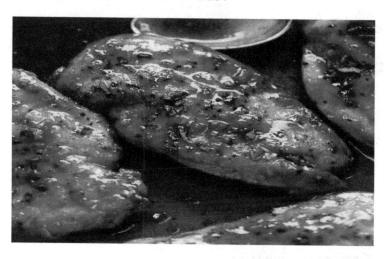

INGREDIENTS

- 2 cups of olive oil
- 4 tablespoons garlic, thinly sliced
- 1 cup of guajillo chili pepper, cut into slices
- 4 chicken breasts
- 1 pinch of salt
- 1 pinch of pepper
- 1/4 cups of parsley, finely chopped, to decorate

PREPARATION

1. For the garlic, in a bowl mix the oil with the garlic, the guajillo chili, the chicken and marinade for 30 minutes. Reservation.
2. Heat a skillet over medium heat, add the chicken with the marinade and cook for about 15 minutes over medium heat or until the garlic is golden brown and the chicken is cooked. Season with salt and pepper. Serve and garnish with chopped parsley.

21. Pork Chicharrón A La Mexicana

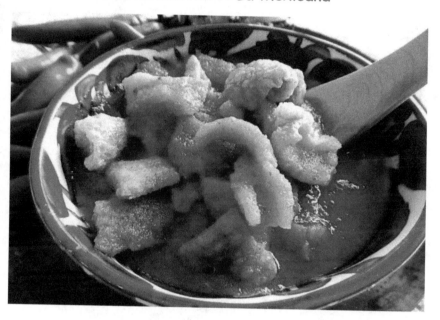

INGREDIENTS

- 1 tablespoon of oil
- 1/4 onions, filleted
- 3 serrano peppers, sliced
- 6 tomatoes, diced
- 1/2 cups of chicken broth
- 3 cups of pork rinds
- enough of salt
- enough of pepper
- enough of fresh coriander, in leaves, to decorate
- enough of beans, from the pot, to accompany

- enough of corn tortillas, to accompany

PREPARATION

1. In a deep frying pan, fry the onion and chili with a little oil until they are shiny. Add the tomato and cook for 5 minutes, add the chicken broth and let it boil. Add the pork rind, season with salt and pepper, cover coriander leaves and cook for 10 minutes.
2. Serve and garnish with coriander leaves.
3. Accompany with pot beans and corn tortillas.

22. Chicken Stuffed With Nopales

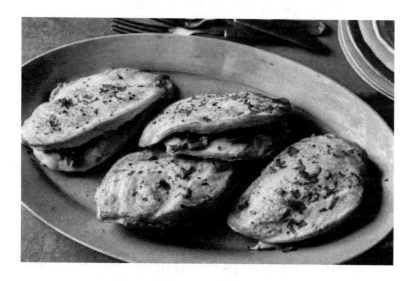

INGREDIENTS

- 1 tablespoon of oil
- 1/2 cups white onion, filleted
- 1 cup of nopal, cut into strips and cooked
- enough of salt
- enough of oregano
- enough of pepper
- 4 chicken breasts, flattened
- 1 cup of Oaxaca cheese, shredded
- 1 tablespoon of oil, for sauce
- 3 cloves of garlic, chopped, for sauce
- 1 white onion, cut in eighths, for sauce
- 6 tomatoes, cut into quarters, for sauce582

- 1/4 cups of fresh coriander, fresh, for sauce
- 4 guajillo chilies, for the sauce
- 1 tablespoon of allspice, for sauce
- 1 Cup of chicken broth, for sauce
- 1 pinch of salt, for sauce

PREPARATION

1. For the filling, heat a pan over medium heat with the oil, cook the onion with the nopales until they stop releasing drool, season to your liking with salt, pepper and oregano. Reservation.

2. On a board, place the chicken breasts, stuffed with the nopales and Oaxaca cheese, roll up, season with salt, pepper and a little oregano. If necessary secure with a toothpick.

3. Heat a grill over high heat and cook the chicken rolls until they are cooked through. Cut the rolls and reserve hot.

4. For the sauce, heat a pan over medium heat with the oil, cook the garlic with the onion until you get a golden color, add the tomato, the coriander, the guajillo chili, the allspice, the coriander seeds. Cook for 10 minutes, fill

with the chicken broth, season with salt, and continue cooking for 10 more minutes. Chill slightly.

5. Blend the sauce until you get a homogeneous mixture. Serve on a plate as a mirror, place the chicken on top and enjoy.

23. Mini Meatloaf With Bacon

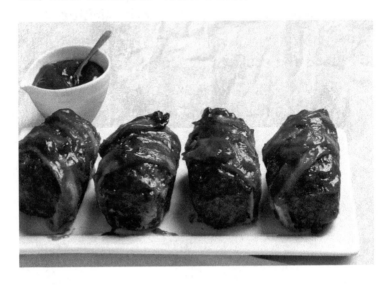

INGREDIENTS

- 1 kilo of ground beef
- 1/2 cups of ground bread
- 1 egg
- 1 cup onion, finely chopped
- 2 tablespoons garlic, finely minced
- 4 tablespoons ketchup
- 1 tablespoon mustard
- 2 teaspoons parsley, finely chopped
- enough of salt
- enough of pepper
- 12 slices of bacon
- enough of ketchup sauce, to varnish
- enough of parsley, to decorate

PREPARATION

1. Preheat the oven to 180 ° C.
2. In a bowl, mix the ground beef with the breadcrumbs, the egg, the onion, the garlic, the ketchup, the mustard, the parsley, the salt and the pepper.
3. Take approximately 150 g of the meat mixture and shape it in a circular shape with the help of your hands. Wrap with bacon and place on a greased cookie sheet or waxed paper. Brush the top of the cupcakes and bacon with ketchup.
4. Bake for 15 minutes or until the meat is cooked and the bacon is golden brown.
5. Serve with parsley, accompanied by salad and pasta.

24. Chicken Wire With Cheese

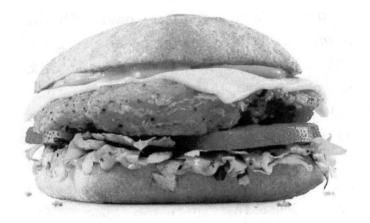

INGREDIENTS

- 1/2 cups chorizo, crumbled
- 1/2 cups bacon, chopped
- 2 tablespoons garlic, finely minced

- 1 red onion, cut into chunks
- 2 chicken breasts, skinless, boneless, diced
- 1 cup mushroom, filleted
- 1 yellow bell pepper, cut into chunks
- 1 red bell pepper, cut into chunks
- 1 bell pepper, orange cut into chunks
- 1 pumpkin, cut into half moons
- 1 pinch of salt and pepper
- 1 cup of Manchego cheese, grated
- to taste of corn tortillas, to accompany
- to taste of sauce, to accompany
- to taste of lemon, to accompany

PREPARATION

1. Heat a skillet over medium heat and fry the chorizo and bacon until golden brown. Add the garlic and onion and cook until transparent. Add the chicken, season with salt and pepper and cook until golden brown.
2. Once the chicken is cooked, add the vegetables one at a time, cooking for a few minutes before adding the next. Finally, add the cheese and cook 5 more minutes so that it melts, rectify the seasoning.
3. Serve the wire very hot accompanied by corn tortillas, salsa and lemon.

25. Keto Taquitos De Arrachera

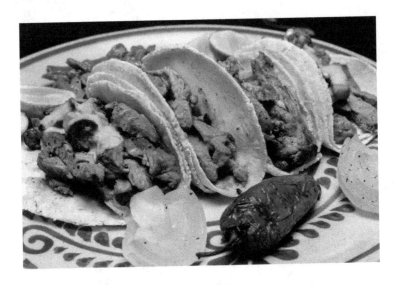

INGREDIENTS

- 3/4 cups of almond flour, 40 g, sifted, for the tortilla
- 1 cup of San Juan® Egg White, 375 ml
- 1 teaspoon of baking powder, 3 g, sifted for the omelette
- to taste of salt, for the omelette
- to taste of pepper, for the omelette
- enough of cooking spray, for the omelette
- 1/4 onions, for the sauce
- 1 clove of garlic, for the sauce
- 1/2 cups of cucumber, without peel or seeds, in cubes, for the sauce
- 2 avocados, just the pulp, for the sauce
- 2 pieces of serrano pepper, without tail, for the sauce
- 3/4 cups of coriander, leaves, for the sauce
- 3 tablespoons of spearmint, leaves, for the sauce
- 3 tablespoons of lemon juice, for the sauce
- 3 tablespoons of Water, for the sauce
- to taste of salt, for the sauce
- to taste of pepper, for the sauce
- 2 tablespoons of olive oil, for the meat
- 1/2 cups of onion, in strips, for the meat
- 500 grams of flank steak, in medium strips
- to taste of salt, for the meat
- to taste of pepper, for the meat
- enough of red onion, pickled, to accompany

- to taste of serrano pepper, sliced, to accompany
- enough of coriander leaf, to accompany

PREPARATION

1. With the help of a balloon, mix the almond flour with the San Juan® Egg White in a bowl and the baking powder until integrated, you will notice that the whites will sponge slightly, season with salt and pepper, and finish integrating.

2. Put a little cooking spray in a Teflon pan (preferably the size you want to make the tortillas) add a little mixture and cook over low heat, when the surface begins to have small bubbles, turn the tortilla with a spatula and cook for a few more minutes. Repeat until finished with the mixture. Reserve hot until use.

3. For the sauce, blend the onion with garlic, cucumber, avocados, serrano pepper, coriander, mint, lemon juice, water, salt, and pepper until integrated. Reserve until use.

4. Pour olive oil into a hot pan, sauté the onion until it is transparent and cook the flank

steak for 8 minutes over medium low heat, season with salt and pepper.

5. Prepare your tacos! Spread sauce on a tortilla, place the flank steak in strips, accompany with pickled onion, serrano slices and cilantro.

26. Keto Mexican Fish Wallpaper

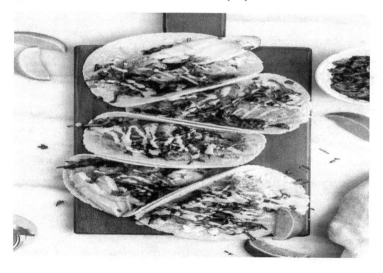

INGREDIENTS

- 4 red snapper fillets, 280 g each
- to taste of garlic powder
- to taste of salt
- to taste of pepper
- 2 bell peppers, cut into strips

- 2 cuaresmeño chile, finely chopped
- enough of epazote, in leaves
- enough of banana leaf, roasted
- 2 pieces of avocado, for the guacamole
- 3 tablespoons of lemon juice, for the guacamole
- 1/4 cups of onion, finely chopped, for the guacamole
- 2 tablespoons of coriander, finely chopped, for the guacamole
- 2 teaspoons of oil

PREPARATION

1. Season the red snapper fillets with the garlic powder, salt and pepper.
2. Place the red snapper fillets on the banana leaves, add the pepper, the cuaresmeño pepper and the epazote leaves.
3. Cover the fish with the banana leaves and wrap as if it were a tamale, place in a steamer and cook for 15 minutes over low heat.
4. In a bowl with the help of a fork, the guacamole mash the avocado until obtaining a puree, add the lemon juice, the onion, season with salt, pepper, add the coriander and mix.
5. Serve on a plate, accompanied by guacamole. Enjoy.

27. Low Carb Chicken Tacos

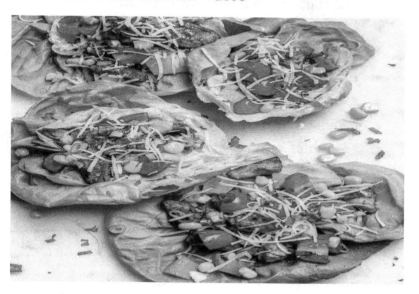

INGREDIENTS

- 1/2 cups pumpkin, Italian, sliced
- 1 cup of almond flour
- 2 tablespoons cornstarch
- 4 eggs
- 1 1/2 cups of milk
- to taste of salt
- enough of Nutrioli® spray oil, for the tortillas
- enough of Nutrioli® spray oil, for sautéing the fajitas

- 1 cup onion, diced
- 2 cups chicken, cubed
- 1/2 cups green bell pepper, diced
- 1/2 cups red bell pepper, diced
- 1/2 cups yellow bell pepper, diced
- 1 cup of Manchego cheese, grated
- enough of coriander, to decorate
- enough of lemon, to accompany
- enough of green sauce, to accompany

PREPARATION

1. Blend the pumpkin, almond flour, cornstarch, egg, milk, and salt.
2. In a non-stick frying pan add the Nutrioli® Spray Oil and with the help of a spoon, shape the tortillas. Cook 3 minutes on each side. Reservation.
3. In a frying pan over medium heat add the Nutrioli® Spray Oil, the onion, the chicken, the salt and the pepper. and cook for 10 minutes.
4. Add the peppers and cook for 5 minutes; add the cheese and cook until melted.
5. Form the tacos, decorate with cilantro and serve with lemon and green sauce.

28. Quinoa Yakimeshi

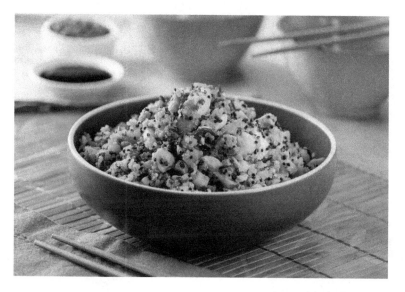

INGREDIENTS

- 1 cup Goya organic tricolor quinoa
- 1 1/2 cups of water
- to taste of salt
- 1 tablespoon of olive oil
- 1 tablespoon chives
- 1 tablespoon of onion
- 1/2 cups of carrot
- 1/2 cups of pumpkin
- 1 1/2 cups of chicken
- 1 egg
- 1/4 cups soy sauce
- enough of chives, to decorate

PREPARATION

1. In a small pot add the Goya tricolor organic Quinoa, the water and the salt. Cover and cook over low heat for 20 minutes. Reservation.
2. In a deep-frying pan add the olive oil, add the onion, chives, carrot and pumpkin. Add the chicken and cook for 10 minutes.
3. Make a circle in the center of the pan and pour in the egg, mix until cooked and integrated.
4. Add the Goya tricolor organic Quinoa, the soy sauce and mix.
5. Garnish with chives and serve hot.

29. Cucumber Rolls Stuffed With Tuna Salad

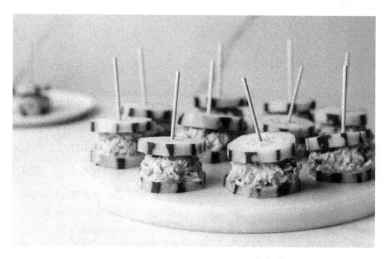

INGREDIENTS

- 1 cucumber
- 1 cup canned tuna, drained
- 1 avocado, diced
- 1/4 cups mayonnaise
- 1 tablespoon of lemon juice
- 1/4 cups of celery
- 2 tablespoons ground chipotle chile
- 1 cuaresmeño pepper, finely chopped
- enough of salt
- enough of pepper

PREPARATION

1. With the help of a peeler, cut the cucumber and remove thin slices.
2. Mix the tuna with the avocado, the mayonnaise, the lemon juice, the celery, the ground chipotle, the cuaresmeño pepper, and season with salt and pepper.
3. Place some tuna on one of the cucumber slats, roll up and repeat with all the others. Serve and decorate with cuaresmeño pepper.

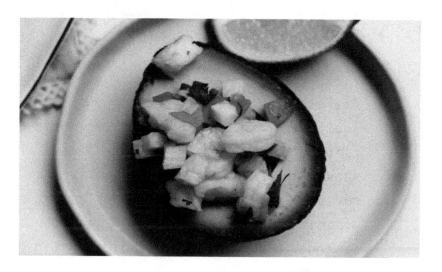

INGREDIENTS

- 400 grams of white fish, cut into cubes
- 1/2 cups of lemon juice
- 1/4 cups of orange juice
- 1/2 tablespoons olive oil
- 1 cucumber, with peel, diced
- 2 tomatillos, diced
- 1 tomato, diced
- 2 habanero peppers, finely chopped
- 1/4 red onions, finely chopped
- 1/2 cups pineapple, diced
- 1/4 cups fresh cilantro, finely chopped
- 1 tablespoon apple cider vinegar
- 1/2 teaspoons of salt

- 1 teaspoon white pepper, ground
- 2 Avocado from Mexico
- 1 radish, thinly sliced, for garnish

PREPARATION

1. In a bowl, marinate the fish with the lemon juice, orange juice and olive oil, refrigerate for about 20 minutes.
2. Remove the fish from the refrigerator and mix with the cucumber, tomatillo, tomato, habanero pepper, red onion, pineapple, coriander, apple cider vinegar and season with salt and white pepper.
3. Cut the avocados in half, remove the seed and the skin, fill each half with the ceviche and decorate with radishes.

31. Keto Chocolate Cake

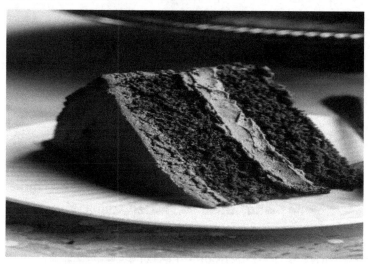

INGREDIENTS

- 10 eggs
- 1 1/4 cups monk fruit
- 1 cup coconut flour
- 1 cup of cocoa
- 1/2 cups of coconut milk
- 1 tablespoon of baking soda
- 1 tablespoon of baking powder
- 1 cup dark chocolate, melted
- 1/2 cups coconut oil, melted
- enough of coconut oil, to grease
- enough of cocoa, for the mold
- 1/2 cups of coconut milk
- 1 cup of dark chocolate

- 1 Cup of almond, filleted, to decorate
- 1 cup of raspberry, to decorate
- enough of chocolate, in shavings, to decorate

PREPARATION

1. Preheat the oven to 170 ° C.
2. In a blender bowl, beat the eggs with the monkfruit until they double in size, gradually add the coconut flour, cocoa, coconut milk, baking soda, baking powder, dark chocolate and oil. coconut. Beat until incorporated and have a homogeneous mixture.
3. Grease a cake pan with the coconut oil and sprinkle with cocoa.
4. Pour in cake mix and bake 35 minutes or until toothpick inserted comes out clean. Let cool and unmold.
5. Heat the coconut milk in a pot over medium heat for the bitumen, add the dark chocolate, and stir until completely melted. Refrigerate and reserve.
6. Beat the frosting until it doubles in size.
7. Cover the cake with the bitumen, decorate with toasted almonds, raspberries and chocolate shavings.
8. Cut a slice and enjoy.

32. Marielle Henaine

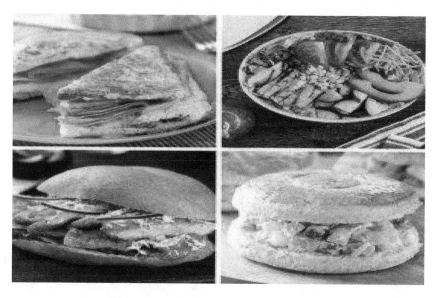

INGREDIENTS

- enough of water
- enough of salt
- 2 cups cauliflower, cut into small pieces
- 1 cup cream cheese
- 1/3 cups of butter
- 1 tablespoon of oregano
- enough of salt
- enough of white pepper
- enough of chives

PREPARATION

1. In a pot with boiling water add the salt and cauliflower, cook until smooth. Drain and chill.
2. Place the cauliflower, cream cheese, butter, salt, and pepper in the processor. Process until you get a very smooth puree.
3. Cook the puree in a pan over medium heat to thicken, correct seasoning and serve with chopped chives.

33. Chayotes Stuffed With Salpicón

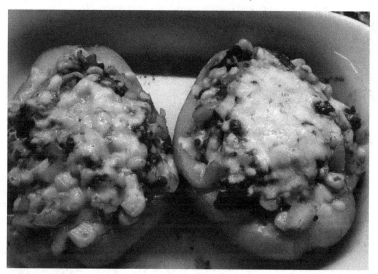

INGREDIENTS

- enough of water
- 1 pinch of salt
- 2 chayotes, peeled and halved
- 1 1/2 cups of beef brisket, cooked and shredded
- 1/4 cups red onion, finely chopped
- 2 green tomatoes, diced
- 2 pickled serrano peppers, sliced
- 1 cup lettuce, finely chopped
- 1 tablespoon oregano, dried
- 1/4 cups lemon juice
- 2 tablespoons olive oil

- 1 tablespoon of white vinegar
- pinches of salt
- enough of pepper
- 1/2 avocados, sliced

PREPARATION

1. In a pot with boiling water and salt, cook the chayotes until soft, about 15 minutes. Remove, drain and reserve.
2. On a board and with the help of a spoon, hollow out the chayote and finely chop the filling.
3. For the salpicón, in a bowl mix the shredded meat with the purple onion, green tomato, serrano pepper, lettuce, coriander, oregano, lemon juice, olive oil, vinegar, chayote filling the salt and the pepper.
4. Fill the chayotes with the salpicón and decorate with avocado.

34. Chicken Broth With Cauliflower Rice

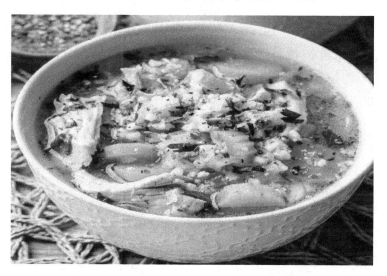

INGREDIENTS

- 2 liters of water
- 1 chicken breast, bone-in and skinless
- 1 clove garlic
- 2 bay leaves
- enough of salt
- 1 cauliflower, cut into small pieces
- 2 chayotes, shelled and diced
- 2 pumpkins, diced
- 2 serrano peppers, finely chopped
- enough of avocado, sliced, to serve
- enough of fresh coriander, finely chopped, to serve
- enough of lemon, to serve

PREPARATION

1. For the broth, heat the water in a pot and cook the chicken breast with the garlic, bay leaf and salt. Cover and boil until the breast is cooked, about 40 minutes.

2. Remove the chicken breast, cool and shred. Strain the chicken broth to remove impurities and fat.

3. Blend the cauliflower in a food processor until very small pieces have a "rice" consistency.

4. Return the broth to cooking covered, once it boils, add the chayotes and cook for a few minutes without uncovering the pot. Add the pumpkins and the serrano pepper, cook until soft. Once the vegetables are cooked, add the cauliflower and chicken, cook 5 more minutes and season.

5. Serve the chicken broth with avocado, cilantro and a few drops of lemon.

35. Coleslaw And Chicken

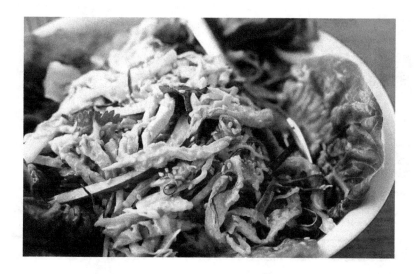

INGREDIENTS

- 1 chicken breast, cooked and shredded
- 1 cup white cabbage, cut into strips
- 1 cup of mayonnaise
- 2 tablespoons mustard
- 1 tablespoon of white vinegar
- enough of salt
- enough of pepper

PREPARATION

1. In a bowl mix the chicken with the cabbage, mayonnaise, mustard, vinegar, season with salt and pepper.
2. Serve and enjoy.

36. Roasted Chicken With Guajillo

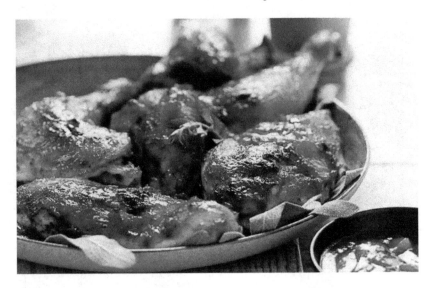

INGREDIENTS

- 2 cloves of garlic
- 7 guajillo chiles, deveined and seeded
- 1 cup butter, at room temperature
- 1 tablespoon onion powder
- 1 tablespoon oregano, dried
- 1 tablespoon of salt
- 1/2 tablespoons of pepper
- 1 chicken, skin on, cleaned and butterfly cut (1.5 kg)

PREPARATION

1. Preheat the oven to 220 ° C.
2. On a comal, roast the garlic and guajillo chiles. Remove and blend until you get a fine powder.
3. In a bowl, mix the butter with the guajillo chili powder and garlic, onion powder, oregano, salt and pepper.
4. Brush the chicken with the butter mixture on all sides, including between the skin and the meat. Place it on a baking sheet and bake for 45 minutes.
5. Remove the chicken from the oven, re-glaze with the butter and lower the oven temperature to 180 ° C.
6. Bake again for 15 more minutes or until cooked through. Remove and serve, accompany with a green salad.

37. Poblano Broccoli Rice

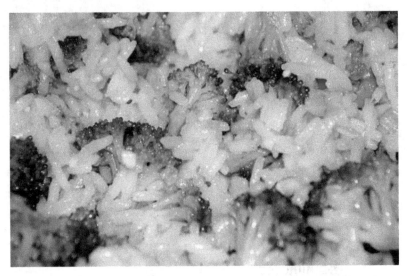

INGREDIENTS

- 1 broccoli, (1 1/2 cup) cut into small pieces
- 1 clove garlic
- 2 poblano peppers, tatemados, sweaty, skinless and seeded
- 1/2 cups of vegetable broth
- 1 tablespoon onion powder
- enough of salt
- 1 tablespoon of oil
- 1 cup of poblano rajas
- enough of fresh coriander, to decorate

PREPARATION

1. Place the broccoli in the processor and mash until it has a "rice" consistency.
2. Blend the garlic with the poblano peppers, the vegetable broth, the onion powder and the salt, until you get a homogeneous mixture.
3. In a saucepan, heat the oil over medium heat and cook the broccoli for a few minutes. Add the previous mixture and the slices, cook over low heat until the liquid is consumed. Rectify seasoning.
4. Serve the rice decorated with coriander.

38. Pumpkins Stuffed With Creamy Chicken Salad

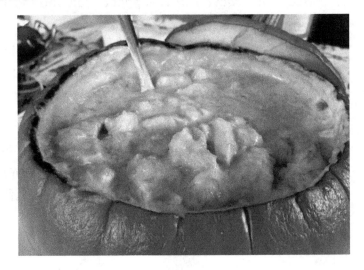

INGREDIENTS

- enough of water
- enough of salt
- 4 green squash, Italian

- 2 cups chicken, cooked and shredded
- 1/3 cups mayonnaise, chili peppers
- 1 tablespoon mustard, yellow
- 1/4 cups fresh cilantro, finely chopped
- 1/2 cups celery, finely chopped
- 1/2 cups of bacon, Fried and chopped
- 1 tablespoon onion powder
- 1/2 tablespoons garlic powder
- enough of salt
- enough of pepper
- enough of fresh coriander, Leaves, to decorate

PREPARATION

1. Heat salted water in a pot, when it boils add the pumpkins and cook for 5 minutes. Drain and chill.
2. For the salad, mix the shredded chicken with the chilli mayonnaise (mix mayonnaise with dried chili powder and you're done), the mustard, the coriander, the celery, the fried bacon , the onion powder, the garlic powder, the salt and pepper.

3. With the help of a knife, cut the tips of the pumpkins, cut in half lengthwise and hollow out with the help of a spoon.
4. Fill the squash with the salad and decorate with fresh cilantro. It serves.

39. Arrachera Salad With Fine Herb Vinaigrette

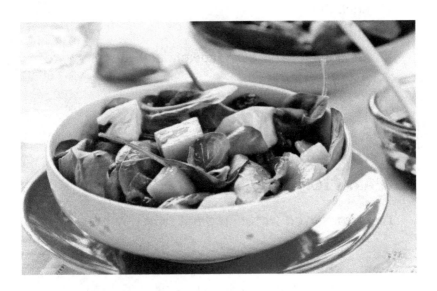

INGREDIENTS

- 400 grams of flank steak, diced
- enough of salt
- enough of pepper
- 1 tablespoon of olive oil

- 3 tablespoons of white vinegar, for the vinaigrette
- 1/2 tablespoons of Dijon mustard, for the vinaigrette
- 1/2 tablespoons of fresh rosemary, for the vinaigrette
- 1/2 tablespoons of dried thyme, for the vinaigrette
- 1/2 tablespoons of dried oregano, for the vinaigrette
- 1/2 cups of olive oil, for the vinaigrette
- 2 cups of mixed lettuce, for the salad
- 1 cup baby spinach
- 1 cup artichoke heart, halved

PREPARATION

1. Season the flank steak with salt and pepper, and cook in a skillet over medium heat with olive oil to the desired finish. Withdraw and reserve.
2. For the vinaigrette, blend the white vinegar with the mustard, rosemary, thyme, oregano, salt and pepper. Without stopping blending, add the olive oil in the form of a thread until

it emulsifies, that is, the mixture is completely integrated.

3. In a bowl, mix the lettuce with the spinach, the artichoke hearts, the flank steak and the vinaigrette. Serve and enjoy.

40. How To Make Chicken Meatballs In Morita Chili Sauce

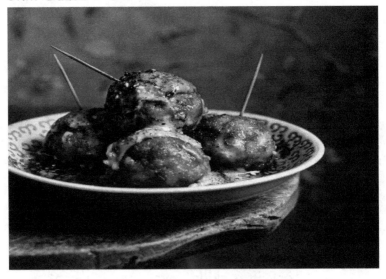

INGREDIENTS

- 500 grams of ground chicken meat
- 1 tablespoon garlic powder
- 1 tablespoon onion powder
- 1 tablespoon parsley, finely chopped
- 1 tablespoon fresh coriander, finely chopped

- enough of salt
- enough of pepper
- olive oil spoons
- 2 cups green tomato, quartered
- 2 cloves of garlic
- 2 morita peppers, deveined and seeded
- 1 cup of chicken broth
- 1 branch of fresh coriander
- 1/4 tablespoon ground cumin, whole
- 1 tablespoon of olive oil
- enough of Chinese parsley, to accompany

PREPARATION

1. Mix the ground chicken meat with the garlic powder, the onion powder, the parsley, the coriander, season with salt and pepper.
2. With the help of your hands, form the meatballs and reserve.
3. Heat the oil over medium heat in a saucepan and fry the tomatoes, garlic and chilies for 5 minutes. Fill with the chicken broth, cilantro and cumin, cook for 5 minutes. Chill slightly.
4. Blend the previous preparation until you get a smooth sauce.
5. Fry the sauce again with a little more oil, cook for 10 minutes over medium heat, add the meatballs, and cover and cook until the meatballs are cooked.

6. Serve the meatballs and garnish with parsley.

41. Crust Stuffed With Meat With Nopales

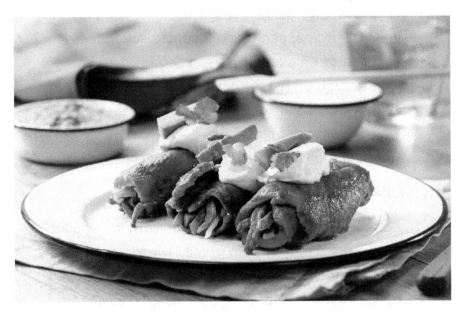

INGREDIENTS

- 1 tablespoon of oil
- 1 cup of nopal, diced
- 500 grams of beef steak, minced
- 1 cup of Manchego cheese, grated
- 1 cup gouda cheese, grated
- 1/2 cups parmesan cheese, grated
- enough of green sauce, to serve
- 1/2 avocados, to serve, sliced

- enough of fresh coriander, fresh, to serve
- enough of lemon, to serve

PREPARATION

1. Heat a pan over medium heat with the oil, add the nopales and cook until they have no babita, then cook the beef steak with the nopales and season with salt and pepper to your liking. Remove from heat.
2. Heat a skillet over high heat and cook the cheeses until a crust forms, remove from the pan and fold into a taco shape, let cool to harden. Repeat until finished with the cheeses.
3. Fill the cheese crusts with the meat and serve with the green sauce, avocado, cilantro and lemon.

42. Pumpkin Spaghetti With Avocado Cream

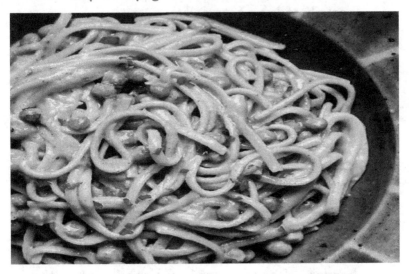

INGREDIENTS

- 2 avocados
- 1/4 cups cilantro, cooked
- 1 tablespoon of lemon juice
- 1 pinch of salt
- 1 pinch of pepper
- 1/2 tablespoons onion powder
- 1 clove garlic
- 1 tablespoon of olive oil
- 4 cups of pumpkin, in noodles
- 1 tablespoon of salt
- 1 tablespoon of pepper
- 1/4 cups of Parmesan cheese

PREPARATION

1. For the sauce, process the avocado with the cilantro, lemon juice, salt, pepper, onion powder and garlic until you get a smooth puree.

2. Heat a pan over medium heat with the oil, cook the pumpkin noodles, season with salt and pepper, add the avocado sauce, mix and cook for 3 minutes, serve with a little Parmesan cheese and enjoy.

43. Cauliflower Omelette With Spinach And Serrano Chile

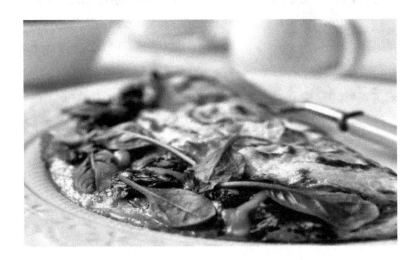

INGREDIENTS

- 1/2 cups of water
- 2 cups of spinach leaf
- 3 serrano peppers
- 1 cup cornmeal
- 4 cups of Cauliflower Eva® Bits, 454 g
- 1 tablespoon garlic powder
- to taste of salt
- to taste of pepper
- enough of chicken tinga, to accompany

PREPARATION

1. Pour the Cauliflower Eva Bits into a pot of hot water. Cook for 4 minutes, drain and cool down under the stream of cold water. Remove the excess water with the help of a cotton cloth. Reserve until use.
2. Blend the spinach, the serrano pepper with a little cold water until you have a pasty mixture. Reserve until use. Strain and reserve the pulp.
3. In a bowl, place the Cauliflower Eva Bits, the garlic powder, the cornmeal, the spinach pulp, salt and pepper, and mix until integrated. With the help of your hands, form balls and reserve.
4. In a tortilla press, place a plastic and press the ball to form the tortilla.
5. On a comal over medium heat cook the tortilla on both sides until lightly golden brown.
6. Accompany your tortilla with chicken tinga.

44. Roasted Cauliflower With Egg And Avocado

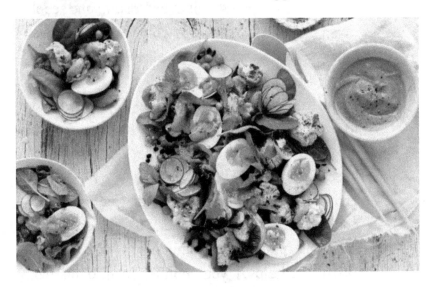

INGREDIENTS

- 1 cauliflower
- 1 tablespoon of olive oil
- 1/4 cups of Parmesan cheese
- 2 tablespoons garlic powder
- 1 tablespoon of salt
- 1 tablespoon of pepper
- 4 eggs
- 1 avocado, cut into wedges
- enough of oregano, fresh

PREPARATION

1. Preheat the oven to 200 ° C.
2. Cut cauliflower slices 1 to 2 fingers thick, place on a baking sheet. Bathe with the olive oil, Parmesan cheese, garlic powder, a little salt and pepper.
3. Bake for 15 minutes or until cauliflower is cooked through and golden brown. Remove from the oven and reserve.
4. Heat a skillet over medium heat and grease with a little cooking spray. Crack an egg and cook to the desired term. Season to your liking.
5. Place a little avocado on each slice of cauliflower, a starry egg, decorate with the oregano, serve and enjoy.

45. Chayote Carpaccio

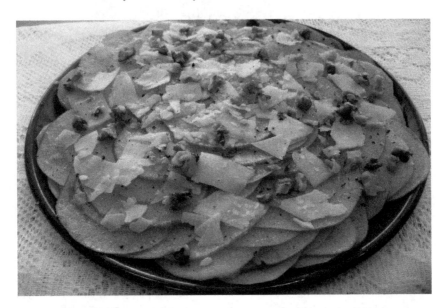

INGREDIENTS

- 4 chayotes
- to taste of salt
- 1/2 cups of basil, for the dressing
- 1/2 cups of mint, for the dressing
- 1/4 cups of yellow lemon juice, for the dressing
- 1/4 cups of olive oil, for the dressing
- 1/2 cups pumpkin, sliced
- 1 teaspoon of chili powder, to decorate
- enough of alfalfa germ, to decorate
- enough of edible flower, to decorate

PREPARATION

1. On a board, peel the chayotes, cut into slices $\frac{1}{2}$ cm thick. Reservation

2. In a pot with water, cook the chayotes for 5 minutes, remove from the heat and drain. Reservation.

3. In a processor add the basil, mint, lemon juice and olive oil, process for 3 minutes. Reservation

4. On a plate, place the chayote slices, season with salt, add the pumpkin slices, the basil and mint dressing, season with the chili powder, decorate with alfalfa germ and edible flowers. Enjoy!

46. Green Cauliflower Enchiladas With Chicken

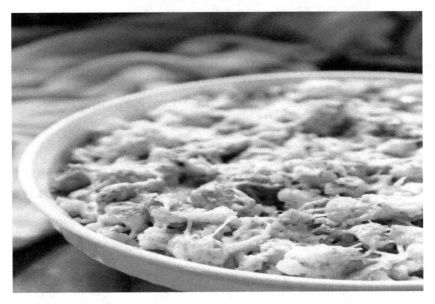

INGREDIENTS

- 4 cups of cauliflower, grated, for the cauliflower tortillas
- 1/2 cups of Chihuahua cheese, low in fat, grated, for the cauliflower tortillas
- 2 eggs, for the cauliflower omelettes
- 5 cups of Water, for the green sauce
- 10 green tomatoes, for the green sauce
- 4 serrano peppers, for the green sauce
- 1/4 onions, for the green sauce
- 1 clove of garlic, for the green sauce
- to taste of salt, for the green sauce
- to taste of pepper, for the green sauce

- 1 tablespoon of olive oil, for the green sauce
- 2 cups chicken breast, cooked and shredded
- enough of Manchego cheese, low in fat, to gratin
- enough of low-fat sour cream, to accompany
- to taste of avocado, to accompany
- to taste of onion, to accompany

PREPARATION

1. In a bowl, place the cauliflower, cover with non-stick plastic, cook 4 minutes in the microwave oven. Strain to remove the water and reserve.
2. Mix the cauliflower with the cheese, eggs, season with salt and pepper and mix until incorporated.
3. Place the cauliflower mixture on a tray lined with wax paper and spread to the size and shape. Bake for 15 minutes at 180 ° C.
4. Fill the tortillas with the shredded chicken and reserve.
5. In a pot with water, cook the tomatoes, serrano peppers, onion, and garlic over medium heat. Let cool, blend and reserve.
6. In a pot over low heat heat the olive oil, pour the sauce, season with salt and pepper and cook for 10 minutes or until it thickens.

7. Serve the enchiladas on an extended plate, bathe with the hot sauce, add the Manchego cheese, microwave for 30 minutes to gratin, decorate with cream, avocado and onion.

47. Sea And Land Keto Skewers

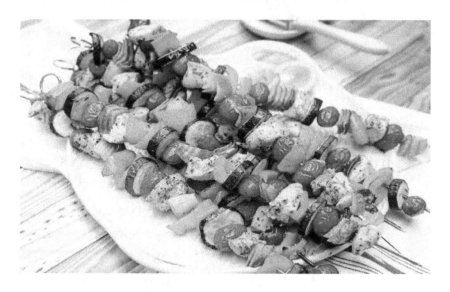

INGREDIENTS

- 1 cup of pumpkin
- 1 cup of red pepper
- 1 cup shrimp, fresh, medium
- 1 cup of yellow bell pepper
- 1 Cup of beef fillet, in medium cubes, for skewer
- 1 cup of green pepper
- enough of cooking spray
- 1 cup of mayonnaise, light
- 1/4 cups coriander
- 1/4 cups of parsley
- 1 tablespoon of lemon juice

- 1 tablespoon garlic powder
- to taste of salt

PREPARATION

1. On a board cut the pumpkin into slices. Similarly, cut the peppers into medium squares and reserve.
2. Insert squash, red bell pepper, shrimp, yellow bell pepper, beef steak, green bell pepper on skewer sticks and repeat until filled.
3. Cook on a grill with a little cooking spray at medium high heat for 15 minutes.
4. For the cilantro dressing: Blend the mayonnaise, cilantro, parsley, lemon juice, garlic powder, and salt until smooth.
5. Serve the skewers with the cilantro dressing and enjoy.

48. Roasted Zucchini With Cottage Cheese

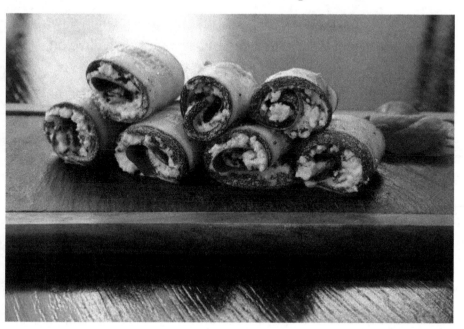

INGREDIENTS

- 3 zucchini, elongated
- 2 tablespoons olive oil
- to taste of salt
- to taste of pepper
- 50 grams of cottage cheese
- 1 tablespoon parsley, minced
- 1/2 teaspoons lemon juice, seeded
- 2 cups baby spinach, leaves
- 1/2 cups basil, leaves

PREPARATION

1. On a board, cut the ends of the zucchini, slice them lengthwise and brush them with olive oil. Season with salt and pepper.
2. On a hot grill over medium heat, place the zucchini slices, grill on both sides for about 5 minutes. Remove from heat and reserve.
3. In a bowl mix the cottage cheese, parsley and lemon juice until integrated.
4. Spread the pumpkin slices on a board, place half a spoon of the previous mixture 2 centimeters from the edge of the pumpkin. Top with baby spinach leaves to taste and add a basil leaf. Roll up.
5. Serve immediately and enjoy.

49. Omelette Poblano

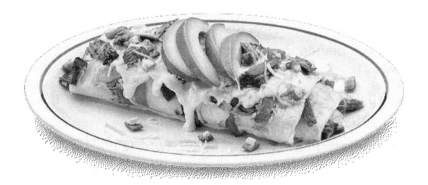

INGREDIENTS

- 1 Cup of poblano pepper, roasted and cut into slices, for the sauce
- 1/4 onions, for the sauce
- 1 clove of garlic, for the sauce
- 1/2 cups of jocoque, for the sauce
- 1 cup of skim milk, light, for the sauce
- to taste of salt, for the sauce
- to taste of pepper, for the sauce
- 1 tablespoon of olive oil, for the sauce
- 4 eggs
- 2 tablespoons skim milk, light
- 1 teaspoon onion powder

- enough of cooking spray
- enough of panela cheese, in cubes, to fill
- enough of red onion, sliced, to accompany

PREPARATION

1. Blend the poblano pepper slices with the onion, garlic, jocoque, skim milk, season with salt and pepper.
2. Heat a pot over medium heat, heat the oil and pour the sauce, cook for 10 minutes, or until it has a thick consistency.
3. For the omelette, in a bowl beat the eggs with the milk, the onion powder, season with salt and pepper. Reservation.
4. In a Teflon pan, add a little olive oil in spray and pour the previous preparation, cook 5 minutes over low heat on each side. Remove from heat and reserve.
5. Fill the omelette with panela cheese, serve on an extended plate, bathe with the poblano sauce, decorate with red onion and enjoy.

50. Egg Cake With Asparagus

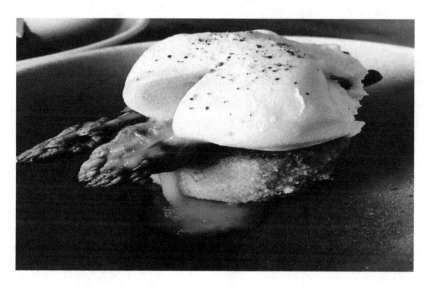

INGREDIENTS

- enough of cooking spray
- 12 egg whites
- 1/2 cups of onion
- 1/2 cups of bell pepper
- 1/2 cups of asparagus
- to taste of salt
- to taste of pepper
- 1/4 teaspoon garlic powder

PREPARATION

1. Preheat the oven to 175 ° C.
2. Spray cupcake pan with a little cooking spray.
3. Add the egg whites, onion, peppers, asparagus, salt, pepper, and garlic powder to a mixer and beat for 5 minutes.
4. Pour the mixture into the cupcake pans, up to $\frac{3}{4}$ percent full, and bake for 20 minutes or until done. Unmold.
5. Serve and enjoy.

51. PRIMITIVE TORTILLA

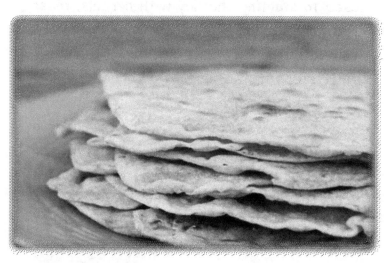

INGREDIENTS

- 1 tablespoon (15 ml) butter with salt
- 30 g chopped mushrooms
- 30 g chopped onion
- 30 g chopped red pepper
- 4 medium eggs
- 30 ml milk cream
- 1/4 tsp (1 ml) salt
- 1/8 teaspoon (0.5 ml) freshly ground pepper
  14 g shredded cheddar cheese (optional)

PREPARATION

1. This is the quintessential primitive breakfast and a fantastic way to gradually abandon the typical carbohydrate breakfast. If you are used to starting the day with cereals, toast and juice, taking a delicious tortilla will keep you satiated for hours and will make your first steps in the paleolithic and ketogenic diet a real pleasure.
2. Melt half the butter over medium heat in a pan. Add the vegetables and sauté them for five to seven minutes. Remove the vegetables from the pan.
3. In the same pan, melt the rest of the butter. In a small bowl, beat the eggs with the cream, salt and pepper. Tilt the pan so that the butter covers the entire bottom. Pour the egg mixture and repeat the movement.
4. Cook without stirring. When the egg sets on the edges, use a Silicone spatula to remove it from the sides of the pan. Tilt the pan so that the egg mixture that occupies the center can reach the edges.
5. When the egg mixture is curdled, put the vegetables on one of the halves of the tortilla. Sprinkle with half the cheese (if used) and carefully fold the tortilla to cover them. Put the tortilla on a plate and sprinkle

with the rest of the cheese. Serve immediately.

52. EGG SALAD FOR BREAKFAST

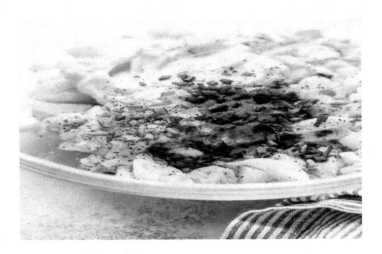

INGREDIENTS

- ½ medium avocado
- 1/3 cup (75 ml) of Primal Kitchen mayonnaise or other mayonnaise suitable for the paleolithic diet (see Note)
- 6 large hard-boiled eggs
- 4 slices of bacon (no added sugar), cooked until crispy
- 2 tablespoons (30 ml) very chopped scallions
- teaspoon (2 ml) tahini (see Note) Freshly ground pepper

PREPARATION

1. This tasty egg salad is fantastic served alone or on a bed of spinach. You can also lightly toast a slice of Keto bread and prepare a sandwich with the salad.
2. In a medium bowl, crush the avocado with a fork. Add the mayonnaise and stir until it forms a homogeneous mass.
3. Chop the hard-boiled eggs. Add them to the mayonnaise mixture and stir everything with a fork, crushing the egg (it should be a little thick).
4. Chop the bacon. Add the pieces, chives and tahini to the egg mixture. Stir. Try and add pepper.

53. COCONUT FLOUR CREPES WITH MACADAMIA NUT

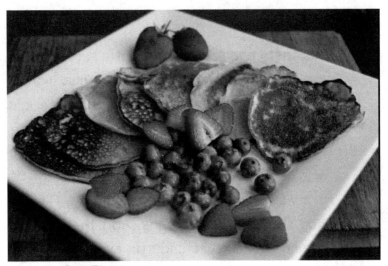

INGREDIENTS

- 3 large eggs
- cup (60 g) butter without melted sugar
- cup (60 g) thick cream
- cup (60 g) whole coconut milk
- teaspoon (2 ml) vanilla extract $\frac{1}{4}$ cup (30 g) coconut flour </
- $\frac{1}{4}$ teaspoon (1 ml) of kosher salt
- teaspoon (2 ml) ground cinnamon
- Sweetener suitable for the ketogenic diet, to taste (optional; see Note)
- cup (30 g) chopped or ground macadamia nuts Coconut oil to grease the grill

PREPARATION

1. Coconut flour crepes are an excellent substitute for those made with white or whole wheat flour. Macadamia nuts add healthy fats and an interesting texture; if you leave them in larger pieces, you will get crunchy crepes. You can replace the thick cream with more coconut milk if you don't want to use dairy products. Serve hot with butter, almond butter, coconut butter or coconut milk cream.
2. In a medium bowl, beat the eggs together with the butter, cream, coconut milk and vanilla.
3. In a small bowl, mix the flour, salt, yeast, cinnamon and sweetener with a fork. Undo lumps and incorporate dry ingredients.
4. Pour the macadamia nuts and stir. The dough will be thick. Add water very little by little until it acquires the desired consistency.
5. Heat a flat-bottomed grill or pan over medium heat. When ready, lightly grease with coconut oil. Put the dough on the grill to large tablespoons. It will be necessary to use a spoon or spatula to spread the dough gently to form a thinner crepe, because its texture will not be that of the traditional dough.

6. Cook slowly, several minutes on each side, until bubbles form. Turn around. Serve hot.

54. HAMBURGER PAN

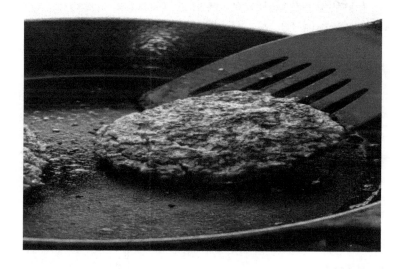

INGREDIENTS

- 900 g of minced beef
- 2 sliced garlic cloves
- 1 teaspoon (5 ml) dried oregano
- 1 teaspoon (5 ml) of kosher salt
- teaspoon (2 ml) black pepper 3 cups (85 g) fresh baby spinach
- 1 ½ cups (170 g) shredded cheese (cheddar or similar) 4 large eggs

PREPARATION

1. I turn to this dish at any time of the day, but especially at breakfast. Feel free to add a couple of pieces of fried bacon to enjoy a cheeseburger and bacon.
2. Preheat the oven to 200 ° C.
3. In a pan suitable for the oven (for example, cast iron), brown the minced meat. After about five minutes, when it is a little done, set it aside and add the garlic. Sauté it for a

minute or so and mix it with the meat. Add oregano, salt and pepper and stir well.

4. Add the handfuls in handful spinach as they soften. As soon as all the spinach is incorporated, remove the pan from the oven. Add

5. cup (120 g) of cheese and stir.

6. Spread the meat evenly in the pan. Next, create four holes in the top of the meat and carefully shell an egg in each. Sprinkle with the rest of the cheese.

7. Bake ten minutes. The whites have to be curdled and the yolks still liquid Leave in the oven a few more minutes to obtain firmer yolks. Serve each serving on a plate.

55. TURNIP HASH BROWNS

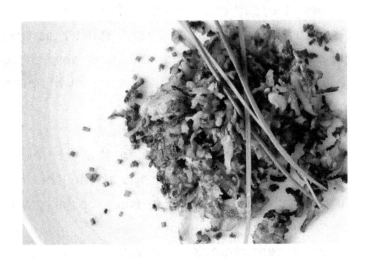

INGREDIENTS

- 2 medium turnips (230 g) washed and peeled
- 1 large egg
- 1 tablespoon (15 ml) coconut flour (optional)
- 1 teaspoon (5 ml) of kosher salt and a little more, to taste ½ teaspoon (2 ml) of black pepper
- 2 tablespoons (30 ml) of bacon or butter fat, or more if necessary
- Sour cream (optional)
- Chopped Chives (optional)

PREPARATION

1. When you have tried these hash browns, the version with potatoes will seem bland in comparison. Serve with a frittata to enjoy a complete ketogenic brunch.
2. Cut the turnips into julienne with a box grater or kitchen robot.
3. Beat the egg in a large bowl and add the turnips. Incorporate stirring the flour, salt and pepper.
4. Heat a large flat-bottomed pan over medium-high heat. Once hot, add the bacon fat; When it has melted, lower the heat a little.
5. Stir the turnips a little more and add them in $\frac{1}{2}$ cup portions (120 ml) approximately in hot fat. Squeeze them a little with a spatula to flatten them. Cook for three to five minutes, until the edges are golden brown. Then, turn around and cook on the other side.
6. Serve on a plate and add a little more salt. If desired, cover with a portion of sour cream and decorate with chives.

56. BOWL OF GREEK YOGURT WITH ALMOND CRISP

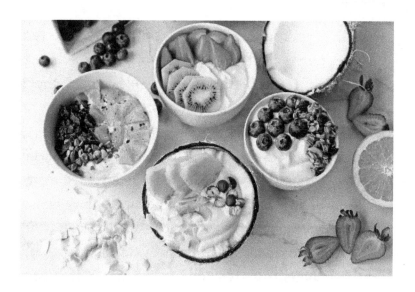

INGREDIENTS

- cup (15 g) unsweetened coconut flakes 2 tablespoons (15 g) filleted almonds
- 1 cup (250 ml) whole Greek yogurt
- 1 / 3 cup (80 ml) of whole coconut milk
- Keto diet sweetener, to taste (optional)
- 2 tablespoons (30 ml) raw almond butter (no added sugar)
- 2 tablespoons (15 g) cocoa beans
- A little ground cinnamon

PREPARATION

1. The cocoa beans are simply the roasted beans of the cocoa plant with which the chocolate is made. But don't expect them to taste the same as your favorite chocolate. They are pure cocoa, that is, unprocessed chocolate, without sugar or other ingredients. Cocoa beans have many health benefits; For example, they are a great source of magnesium, iron and antioxidants. They provide 5 grams of carbohydrates per serving, but 0 of sugar, so it's up to you to decide if you include them in this recipe and, in that case, how much you do.

2. In a small skillet, toast the coconut flakes over medium-low heat and without any fat, until lightly browned. Repeat the operation with the sliced almonds.

3. Mix by stirring yogurt, coconut milk and sweetener, if used. Divide the mixture between two bowls. Add a tablespoon (15 ml) of almond butter to each and stir to amalgamate (nothing happens if everything is mixed). Sprinkle some

roasted coconut, ground almonds, cocoa beans and cinnamon on top.

57. MINCED MEAT, KALE AND GOAT CHEESE FRITTATA

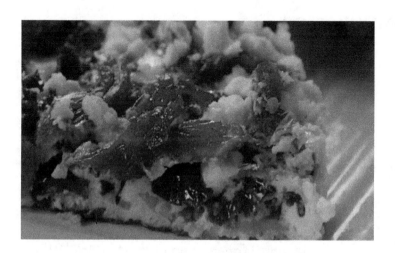

INGREDIENTS

- bunch of kale (4 or 5 leaves), of any variety 1 tablespoon (15 ml) of avocado oil
- 450 g minced pork
- 1 teaspoon (5 ml) dried sage
- 1 teaspoon (5 ml) dried thyme
- ¼ teaspoon (1 ml) ground nutmeg ¼ teaspoon (1 ml) chopped red pepper 1 small onion or ½ large diced
- 2 sliced garlic cloves
- 8 large eggs

- cup (120 ml) thick cream
- 1 cup (90 g) shredded goat cheese, or more, to taste

PREPARATION

1. Every keto diet enthusiast should know how to make a frittata. You can use the combination of meat, cheese, vegetables, herbs and spices that you prefer.
2. With a sharp knife, remove the thick stems of the kale leaves. Cut the stems into dice and chop the leaves. Reserve.
3. Heat the oil over medium heat in a large grill-capable pan (for example, cast iron). When hot, add the pork. Cook for five minutes, stirring occasionally.
4. In a small bowl, mix the sage, thyme, nutmeg and red pepper. Add everything to the meat in the pan and stir well. Continue cooking for another five minutes, until the pork is well done.
5. With a slotted spoon, transfer the meat to a bowl. If there is a lot of fat in the pan, remove a part leaving only one or two tablespoons (15 to 30 ml).

6. Add the onion and kale stalks in the pan. Sauté about five minutes, until the onion softens. Add the garlic and stir for a minute. If necessary, deglaze the pan with a little water, removing the roasted particles.
7. Add the kale leaves handful in handful and stir to soften until all the leaves are in the pan and a little done. Add the meat to the pan and mix well.
8. Beat the eggs with the cream in a medium bowl. Pour the mixture over the meat and vegetables in the pan forming a homogeneous layer. Cook without stirring for about five minutes, until the egg begins to set.
9. Place the oven rack at medium height (about 15 or 20 cm from the top) and turn on the grill. Cover the eggs with goat cheese. Put the pan in the oven and gratin until the egg sets and the goat cheese is lightly toasted. Watch frequently so that it does not burn.
10. Remove the pan from the oven and let it sit for a few minutes. Cut into triangles and serve.

58. BRAD-STYLE KETOAVENA FLAKES

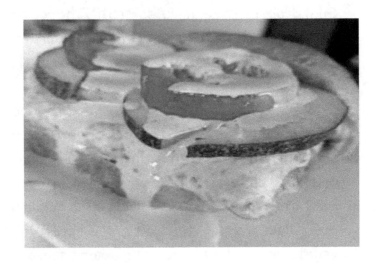

INGREDIENTS

- cup (120 ml) coconut milk 3 egg yolks
- ¼ cup (60 ml) coconut flakes
- teaspoon (2 ml) ground cinnamon

- 1 teaspoon (5 ml) vanilla extract
- cup (60 g) of very ground nuts (nuts, almonds, pecans, macadamia nuts or a mixture)
- 2 tablespoons (30 ml) almond butter
- 1 / 8 teaspoon (0.5 ml) salt (without it if contains almond butter and salt)
- 1 tablespoon (15 ml) cocoa beans (optional)

Coverages

- $\frac{1}{4}$ cup (60 ml) coconut milk
- 2 teaspoons (10 ml) cocoa beans (optional)

PREPARATION

1. This is Brad's response to the detractors of the Keto diet who claim they cannot live without their breakfast cereals. Brad is negotiating with the Ritz-Carlton hotel to add this dish to his healthy breakfast buffet ... Just kidding! Reserve the egg whites to prepare the macarons.

2. Mix the milk and coconut flakes, egg yolks, cinnamon, vanilla, nuts, almond butter, salt and cocoa beans (if used) in a medium saucepan. Heat over medium-low heat, stirring nonstop, for three or four minutes.

3. Serve in two small bowls. Pour in each two tablespoons (30 ml) of coconut milk and a teaspoon of cocoa beans. Eat right away.

59. EGG MUFFINS IN HAM MOLDS

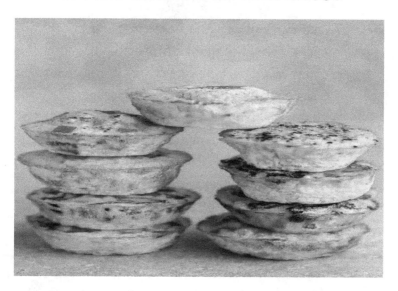

INGREDIENTS

- 1 tablespoon (15 ml) molten coconut oil
- 6 slices of cooked ham (better thinly sliced)
- 6 large eggs
- Salt and pepper to taste
- 3 tablespoons (45 ml) shredded cheddar cheese (optional)

PREPARATION

1. These muffins are the perfect quick breakfast. Prepare them the night before to put one in the microwave or oven the next day. Be sure to buy good quality ham and not cheap sausage.
2. Preheat the oven to 200 ° C. Paint six cavities of a cupcake plate with molten coconut oil.
3. Put a slice of ham and an egg in each cavity. Salpimentar and sprinkle $\frac{1}{2}$ tablespoon (7.5 ml) of cheese on top of each egg.
4. Bake for thirteen to eighteen minutes according to the preferred degree of cooking for egg yolks.
5. Remove the plate from the oven and let it cool for a few minutes before carefully removing the «muffins». Refrigerate in a glass or plastic container so they don't dry out.

60. SPECULOOS, SIMPLIFIED RECIPE

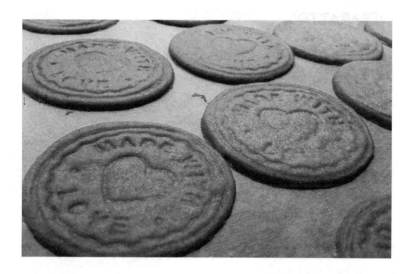

INGREDIENTS

- .250 g butter.
- 350 g flour, sifted.
- 200 g brown sugar
- .5g baking soda.
- 1 egg.
- 1 tablespoon of salt

PREPARATION

9. The preparation of speculoos requires a wait of 12 hours.
10. Mix 40g of flour, baking soda and salt in a first container.
11. Melt the butter.
12. Put it in a second container, add the brown sugar, the egg and mix vigorously. Then add the remaining flour while stirring. Mix everything and let stand 12 hours in the refrigerator.
13. After the 12 hour wait, butter baking sheets.
14. Roll out the dough, keeping a minimum thickness (3 millimeters maximum) and cut it using molds of your choice.
15. Bake everything for 20 minutes, watching the cooking.
16. It is best to let the speculoos cool before eating !

61. CHAI SPICE MIX

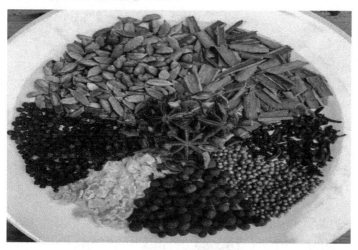

INGREDIENTS

- 2 teaspoons (10 ml) ground cinnamon
- 2 teaspoons (10 ml) ground cardamom
- 1 teaspoon (5 ml) ground ginger
- 1 teaspoon (5 ml) ground cloves
- 1 teaspoon (5 ml) ground allspice

PREPARATION

1. This simple cake can be prepared in advance and only takes a few minutes to assemble. Put it in the fridge and it will be ready in the morning. If you prepare it in small jars with screw cap, you can take them wherever you want. More than you need for this recipe will come out of the spice mixture; Store what you get in an empty spice jar.
2. Mix coconut milk with chia seeds, spice mixture, vanilla and stevia in a bowl (a hand or glass mixer can be used if a more homogeneous texture is preferred).
3. Spread the mixture equally in two jars or small bowls.
4. Refrigerate at least four hours (if possible, overnight), so that it thickens.
5. Add the toppings, if used, and serve.

62. SCRAMBLED EGGS WITH TURMERIC

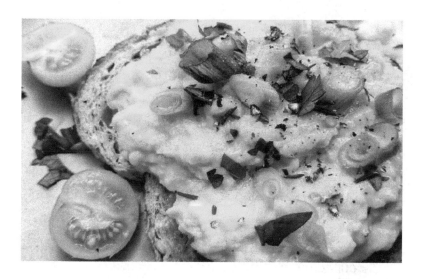

INGREDIENTS

- 3 large eggs
- 2 tablespoons (30 ml) thick cream (optional)
- 1 teaspoon (5 ml) ground turmeric
- Salt to taste
- Freshly ground black pepper to taste
- 1 tablespoon (15 g) of butter

PREPARATION

1. This simple variant of scrambled eggs of a lifetime is a delicious way to start the day and has anti-inflammatory effects. Turmeric is highly prized in health settings because it contains the compound called "curcumin", which has been shown in various studies to be beneficial in numerous ailments, from arthritis to cancer prevention. Do not do without black pepper, because it contains piperine, which improves the absorption of curcumin by the body.

2. In a small bowl, lightly beat the eggs with the cream. Add turmeric, salt and pepper.

3. Melt the butter over medium heat in a pan. When it starts to bubble, gently pour it over the egg mixture. Stir frequently when the eggs begin to set and cook for two or three minutes.

4. Remove from heat, taste, add more salt and pepper if necessary and serve.

63. COCONUT MILK

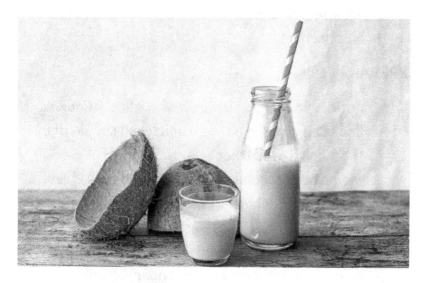

INGREDIENTS

- Coconut milk and ¼ cup of fresh blueberries
- 1 cup (100 g) raw almonds
- 1 cup (100 g) raw cashews
- 1 cup (100 g) raw pumpkin seeds
- 1 cup (100 g) raw sunflower seeds
- cup (60 ml) softened coconut oil 1 tablespoon (15 ml) raw honey
- 1 teaspoon (5 ml) vanilla extract
- 1 teaspoon (5 ml) Himalayan pink salt 1 cup (60 g) unsweetened coconut flakes 1 cup (60 g) cocoa beans

Optional Ingredients

- cup (180 ml) whole coconut milk or unsweetened almond milk ¼ cup (40 g) fresh blueberries

PREPARATION

1. Katie French, author of Paleo Cooking Bootcamp, has created a quick and simple dish that can return cereals to your life. Serve with whole coconut milk or almond milk, fresh berries and whole Greek yogurt, or put the granola in snack bags and take it around.
2. Preheat the oven to 180 ° C. Cover the plate or an iron pot with baking paper.
3. If desired, chop the nuts and seeds with a kitchen robot, a manual chopper or a sharp knife.
4. In a large bowl, mix coconut oil, honey and vanilla. Add the nuts and seeds, sea salt, coconut flakes and cocoa beans and stir well.
5. Move the granola mixture to the baking dish. Bake twenty minutes, turning once, until lightly toasted.
6. Allow the mixture to cool for half an hour and transfer it to an airtight container. Keep it in the fridge for up to three weeks.
7. Add the preferred optional ingredients.

64. CURLEY EGG SNACKS

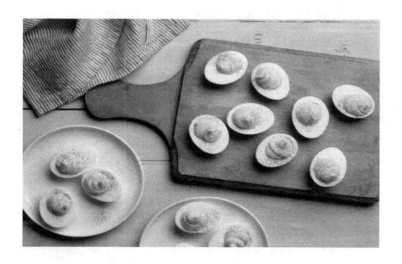

INGREDIENTS

- 1 tablespoon (15 ml) coconut oil
- $\frac{1}{4}$ very chopped onion
- 250 g minced beef raised with grass
- 1 clove garlic fillet
- 1 teaspoon (5 ml) ground cumin
- 1 teaspoon (5 ml) of kosher salt
- $\frac{1}{2}$ teaspoon (2 ml) black pepper
- teaspoon (1 ml) cayenne (optional) 6 large eggs
- $\frac{1}{2}$ cup (45 g) of shredded assorted cheeses

PREPARATION

1. Egg snacks fed a decade of travel around the world of Tyler and Connor Curley, Brad's old friends.

2. Preheat the oven to 200 ° C. Cover a 15 cm square dish with baking paper (or grease well with a tablespoon [15 ml] of molten coconut oil).

3. Heat the oil in a large pan and sauté the onion for a few minutes until it begins to brown.

4. Add the minced meat, stir well and cook for about ten minutes, until you lose almost all the pink hue.

5. Push the minced meat and onion towards the edges of the pan. Put the garlic in the center and cook it until it releases its aroma. Mix everything very well.

6. Add cumin, salt, pepper and cayenne (if used). Stir well and continue cooking for another five minutes, until the meat is completely cooked. Remove from the fire.

7. In a large bowl, beat the eggs. Add a cup of the meat mixture to the eggs, stirring non-stop so that they do not finish curdling. Add the rest of the meat and stir well.

8. Pour the egg and meat mixture into the baking dish. Sprinkle the cheese on top and cook for twenty minutes. Insert a butter

knife in the center; When it comes out clean, remove from the oven. Let it cool for a few minutes and cut into bite-sized squares.

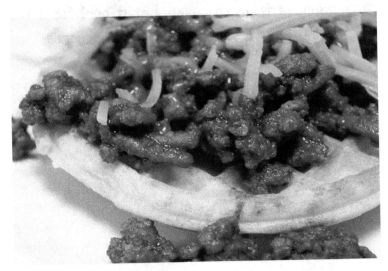

INGREDIENTS

Meat Sauce

- 450 g minced pork (or beef or turkey)
- 1 teaspoon (5 ml) dried sage
- teaspoon (2 ml) dried thyme
- teaspoon (2 ml) ground garlic
- ¼ teaspoon (1 ml) of kosher salt
- ¼ teaspoon (1 ml) of black pepper 300 ml of whole coconut milk (see Note)

Waffles

- 2 large eggs
- 1 tablespoon (15 ml) of molten coconut oil ½ cup (120 ml) of whole coconut milk

- cup (80 g) almond flour or dried fruit pulp (see Note) ¼ teaspoon (1 ml) salt
- ½ teaspoon (2 ml) yeast
- 1½ teaspoons (7 ml) arrowroot powder

PREPARATION

1. This recipe represents a good way to take advantage of the pulp that remains after making dried fruit milk. I prefer to take the time to prepare my own meat sauce starting from scratch, but purchased sausages can be used provided they contain no added sugar or other unacceptable ingredients.

2. Heat a large skillet over medium heat and add the minced meat. Crumble with a fork while cooking.

3. After about five minutes, when the pork is almost done, add the spices and stir well. Stew another two or three minutes, until golden brown. Add coconut milk and wait for it to boil. When that happens, lower the heat.

4. In a medium bowl, beat the eggs with coconut oil and coconut milk. Add the pulp, salt, yeast and arrowroot powder. Mix well. The waffle dough will be thicker than the traditional one; if necessary, add a little water from tablespoon to tablespoon until it acquires the appropriate texture.

5. Pour a little dough into a waffle maker at medium-low heat (you can also use a lightly greased pan or grill and make crepes). Remove the waffle when done and repeat with the rest of the dough.
6. Serve the waffles covered in sauce.

66. HIGH FAT COFFEE

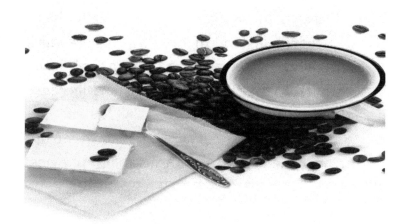

INGREDIENTS

- 1 cup (250 ml) of good quality coffee
- 1-2 tablespoons (15 to 30 ml) unsalted butter
- 1-2 tablespoons (15 to 30 ml) of MCT oil (or coconut oil, although MCT is preferable)

Optional Ingredients

- ½ teaspoon (2 ml) vanilla extract
- teaspoon (1 ml) unsweetened black cocoa powder 1 tablespoon (15 ml) collagen hydrolyzate powder
- A pinch of ground cinnamon

PREPARATION

1. If you used to have a coffee with sugar every morning, you will not miss it once you start enjoying this coffee, full of delicious fats that encourage ketone production. Many adherents of the ketogenic diet drink high-fat coffee instead of breakfast and endure until lunch or dinner. Start with a tablespoon of butter and another MCT oil and increase the dose at your own pace.
2. Beat the coffee, butter and oil with a glass or hand blender until it forms foam. To drink.

67. Ketogenic Protein Mocha

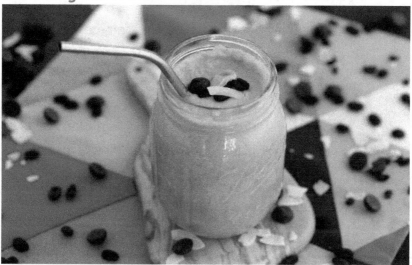

INGREDIENTS

- cup (120 ml) of strong coffee or 1 dose of espresso 1 tablespoon (15 ml) unsalted butter
- 1 tablespoon (15 ml) MCT oil (or coconut oil, although it is preferable to use MCT)
- $\frac{1}{4}$ cup (60 ml) whole, heated or vaporized coconut milk
- 1 scoop (20 g) of Chocolate Coconut Primal Fuel powder meal replacement
- $\frac{1}{4}$ teaspoon (1 ml) unsweetened cocoa powder Hot water
- A pinch of ground cinnamon
- Whipped cream or coconut milk cream (optional)

PREPARATION

1. Try this after a morning training session or when you crave a very expensive sugar bomb from the corner cafeteria.
2. Mix coffee, butter, oil, coconut milk, protein powder and cocoa powder with a glass or arm mixer until it foams. If the drink is too thick, add a little hot water from tablespoon to tablespoon until you get the desired consistency.
3. Pour into a hot cup and sprinkle with a pinch of cinnamon. If desired, add some whipped cream.

68. GREEN SMOOTHIE

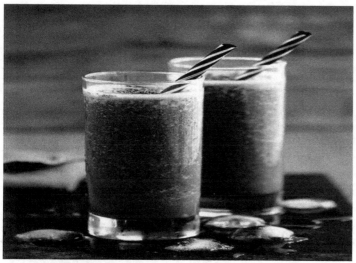

INGREDIENTS

- 1 can (400 ml) whole coconut milk
- 1 teaspoon (5 ml) vanilla extract
- A large bunch of vegetables, such as kale or spinach (about 2 cups)
- 1 tablespoon (15 ml) MCT oil or coconut oil
- 2 / 3 cup (150 g) of crushed ice
- 2 scoops (42 g) of the Primal Fuel (Vanilla Coconut) powder meal replacement

PREPARATION

1. Chocolate Coconut; or normal whey protein powder.
2. When you only have one minute, this option is fantastic and simple.
3. Do not miss the opportunity to take an abundant ration of vegetables.
4. Beat the coconut milk, vanilla, vegetables, oil and ice in a glass blender.
5. Add the protein powder and mix at low power until incorporated. To serve.

69. BEET AND GINGER SMOOTHIE

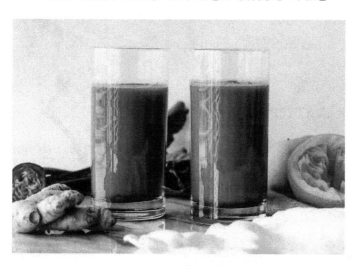

INGREDIENTS

- medium beet (roasted beet is easier to beat; if it is raw, it must first be diced)
- $\frac{1}{4}$ cup (110 g) blueberries, fresh or frozen
- 1 cup (250 ml) almond milk or other unsweetened dried vegetable milk
- A large bunch of vegetables, such as kale or spinach (about 2 cups) 10 macadamia nuts
- A 3 cm piece of fresh ginger peeled and diced 2 tablespoons (30 ml) MCT oil or coconut oil

5-10 drops of liquid stevia, or to taste (optional)

- 2/3 cup (150 g) crushed ice

PREPARATION

1. This smoothie is full of antioxidants, vitamins and minerals, which makes it a fantastic drink to recover in those days when you have trained very intensely. In addition, macadamia nuts and MCT oil provide a good amount of healthy fats.
2. Beat the beets, cranberries, almond milk, vegetables, macadamia nuts, ginger, oil and stevia in a glass blender. A second cycle may be necessary if raw beets are used or if macadamia nuts are not whipped at all.
3. Add the ice and beat everything until the mixture is homogeneous.

70. SMOOTHIE OF WHATEVER

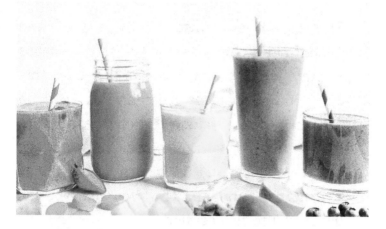

INGREDIENTS

- 3 cups (50 g) kale leaves
- cup (120 ml) whole coconut milk
- medium avocado (approximately ¼ cup; 60 g) ¼ cup (30 g) raw almonds
- 3 Brazil nuts
- cup (30 g) of fresh herbs (see Note)
- 2 scoops of the Chocolate Coconut Primal Fuel powder substitute or normal whey protein powder
- 1 tablespoon (15 ml) cocoa powder (if possible, dark chocolate)
- 1 teaspoon (5 ml) ground cinnamon
- 1 teaspoon (5 ml) Himalayan pink salt
- 2 or 3 drops of peppermint extract (optional)
- 1 or 2 cups of ice cubes

PREPARTION

1. This smoothie is inspired by one of Ben Greenfield's favorite breakfasts, famous triathlete and coach. I call it the "smoothie of whatever" because you can put everything you have in the fridge! Do not hesitate to adapt this recipe to include the nuts and herbs you have. It is a real meal full of calories and nutrients, so, if you wish, you can divide it into two portions.

2. Place a basket for steaming in a small casserole with 2 or 3 cm of water in the bottom. Bring the water to a boil and steam the kale for five minutes.

3. Put the kale in a blender. Add coconut milk, avocado, nuts and herbs. Beat at full power for thirty seconds.

4. Add protein powder, cocoa powder, cinnamon, salt, extract of peppermint and ice, and beat until you get a homogeneous texture.

5. Add water if necessary to obtain the desired consistency.

71. GOLDEN CHAI

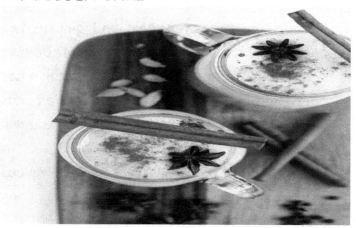

INGREDIENTS

- 1½ cups (375 ml) dried fruit milk
- 1 teaspoon (5 ml) ground turmeric
- 1 teaspoon (5 ml) of chai spice mix
- teaspoon (2 ml) black pepper
- teaspoon (2 ml) vanilla extract
- 1 tablespoon (15 ml) coconut oil or MCT oil
- 1 tablespoon (15 ml) collagen powder (optional)
- 5-10 drops of liquid stevia, or to taste

PREPARATION

1. Since it contains turmeric and ginger, two anti-inflammatory spices, many people believe that golden milk or golden milk has therapeutic properties. This version has added the classic chai spices. A hot cup will help you relax at night.
2. Heat the milk of nuts, turmeric, chai spices and pepper in a saucepan without boiling. Cook slowly for a few minutes.
3. Incorporate vanilla, coconut oil, collagen powder (if used) and stevia.
4. With a hand blender, mix well until it forms foam. Taste and adjust the sweetness with stevia (without overdoing it).

72. Chicken Bone Broth

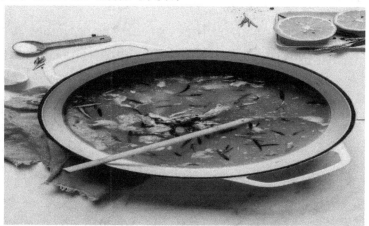

INGREDIENTS

- 4 cups (300 to 400 g) of chicken bones or carcasses of a 1.4 kg chicken
- 2 or 3 cups (150 to 300 g) of vegetable remains (see Council); or 1 large diced onion, with skin and root if it is organically grown, 2 celery sticks and 2 diced carrots, including 2 crushed garlic cloves
- 1 tablespoon (15 ml) sliced fresh ginger
- 10 black peppercorns
- 1 bay leaf
- Fresh herbs, such as thyme or rosemary (optional)

PREPARATION

1. Method 1: Put the bones, the remains of vegetables, garlic, ginger, pepper and bay leaf in a large pot with enough water to cover all the ingredients. Bring to a boil and, when it breaks to a boil, lower the temperature to simmer. Cook for several hours, the longer the better, monitoring the water level and adding more liquid if it drops too low.

2. Method 2: Put the ingredients in a slow cooker with enough water to cover them well. Cover and regulate heat to a minimum. Let it cook for at least eight hours, although the result will be better if it cooks longer. You can cook the broth for twenty-four hours or more.

3. Method 3: Put all the ingredients in an Instant Pot or similar electric pressure cooker and fill it with water (without exceeding the maximum marking line). Close the lid and cook for two hours. Let the pressure rise naturally before opening the pot.

4. When the broth is done, strain with a fine mesh strainer and cool quickly. The easiest way to do this is to put the plug on the sink and fill it with ice water halfway up. Put a

metal bowl or a clean metal pot in the ice water and pour the broth through the strainer.

5. When the broth is cold, transfer it to clean containers (for example, glass jars with screw caps) and put it in the fridge, or freeze it if you do not plan to use it in a couple of days.

73. NUT MILK

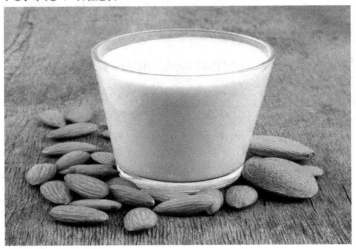

INGREDIENTS

- 1 cup (100 g) of raw nuts (almonds, hazelnuts, cashews, pecans or macadamia nuts)
- 4 cups (1 l) of filtered water plus an additional amount for soaking
- 1 teaspoon (5 ml) vanilla extract (optional)
- $\frac{1}{4}$ teaspoon (1 ml) of salt (optional)
- teaspoon (2 ml) ground cinnamon (optional) Keto diet sweetener, to taste (optional)

PREPARATION

1. This milk is delicious and can be a fantastic option for ketogenic diet enthusiasts who want to avoid eating many dairy products. However, commercial nut milks often contain unacceptable ingredients and sweeteners. Luckily, making it is very easy and you can use the nuts you have on hand.

2. Put the nuts in a glass bowl or jar and cover them completely with filtered water. Let them sit at room temperature for at least four hours, although it will be better to have them eight hours or overnight (up to twenty-four hours).

3. Drain and wash the nuts. Put them in the blender glass and beat them at maximum power with four cups of filtered water to form a homogeneous paste.

4. Strain through a thin cloth or a clean dishcloth. Squeeze the pulp to remove as much milk as possible (see Tip).

5. If you decide to add any of the optional ingredients, rinse the glass, pour the milk and optional ingredients and beat until you get a homogeneous texture.

6. Transfer the dried milk to an airtight container and store it in the fridge. It will last five days.

74. LOW FAT MAC AND CHEESE

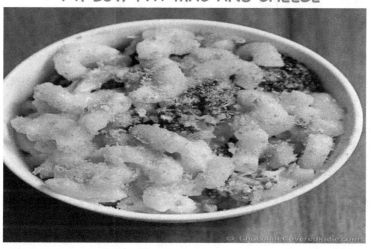

INGREDIENTS

- .1 1/2 t. of macaroni cooked and drained.
- 1 small onion, chopped.
- 9 slices, 2/3 oz strong low fat cheddar cheese.
- 1 12 oz can of evaporated skim milk.
- 1/2 t. low sodium chicken broth.
- 2 1/2 tablespoon (s) tablespoon of flour of wheat around
- .1/4 teaspoon worcestershire sauce.
- 1/2 teaspoon dry mustard.
- 1/8 teaspoon (s) of pepper.
- 3 tablespoon (s) of breadcrumbs.
- 1 tablespoon (s) of margarine, softened

PREPARATION

2. In a deep baking dish sprayed with vegetable oil spray, spread 1/3 of the macaroni, 1/2 of the onions and cheese. Repeat layers, ending with macaroni. Whisk milk, broth, flour, mustard, Worcestershire sauce and pepper until combined. Pour over the layers. Combine breadcrumbs and margarine, then sprinkle on top. Bake uncovered at 375 degrees for 30 minutes until hot and bubbling.

75. FAKE PEANUT SAUCE

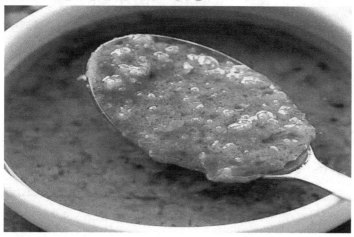

INGREDIENTS

- cup (120 g) raw almond butter
- cup (120 g) whole coconut milk
- 2 large sliced garlic cloves
- The juice of 1 small lime
- 2 tablespoons (30 ml) tamari (gluten-free soy sauce)
- 1 tablespoon (15 ml) grated fresh ginger
- tablespoon (8 ml) roasted sesame oil (see Note)
- tablespoon (8 ml) avocado oil
- $\frac{1}{4}$ teaspoon (1 ml) chopped red pepper (optional)

PREPARATION

1. I love peanut sauce for vegetables, chicken and prawns. However, many enthusiasts of paleolithic and ketogenic diets try to avoid peanuts due to allergy problems since they are technically a legume, not a dried fruit. In addition, they provide more carbohydrates than any dried fruit or seed. Luckily, this peanut sauce prepared with almond butter is as good as the original and has no added sweeteners. Try not to eat it all in one sitting!

2. Mix all the ingredients in a medium bowl or use a small kitchen robot or a hand mixer. Store in the refrigerator in an airtight container. It will last two or three days.

76. PRIMAL KITCHEN MAYONNAISE DRESSING AND BLUE CHEESE

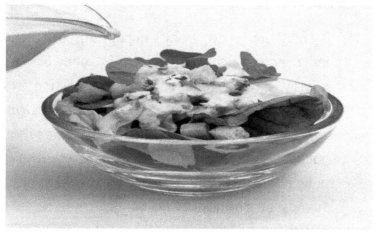

INGREDIENTS

- cup (120 g) of Primal Kitchen mayonnaise ½ lemon juice
- ¼ cup (60 ml) whole coconut milk or thick cream
- ¼ teaspoon (1 ml) of black pepper, or more if ¼ cup (60 ml) of crumbled blue cheese is needed
- Salt (optional)

PREPARATION

1. I may not be very impartial, but the mayonnaise Primal Kitchen is one of my pantry's favorite products. In addition, its intense flavor is perfect for this recipe. You can also use homemade mayonnaise or other packaged mayonnaise if you find any without polyunsaturated oils, although you may have to adjust the flavoring to get the desired flavor.
2. With a whisk of rods, mix the mayonnaise, lemon juice, coconut milk and pepper.
3. Add the blue cheese and stir well. Try and add salt and more pepper if desired.

77. PERFECT VINAIGRETTE (WITH VARIANTS)

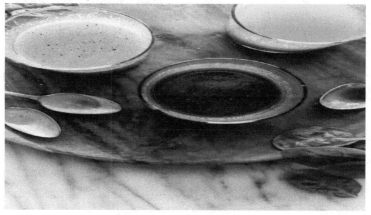

INGREDIENTS

- 1 small shallot very chopped
- 3 tablespoons (45 ml) cider vinegar
- teaspoon (1 ml) kosher salt
- teaspoon (1 ml) black pepper ½ teaspoon (2 ml) Dijon mustard
- ¾ cup (180 ml) extra virgin olive oil

PREPARATION

1. Almost all industrial salad dressings contain polyunsaturated oils that promote inflammation. Luckily, preparing them at home is quick and easy, and represents a great way to add healthy fats to a meal.
2. In a small jar with a lid, mix the shallot, vinegar, salt and pepper.
3. Add mustard and olive oil. Close the bottle tightly and shake vigorously.

Variants

- Lemon Vinaigrette: replace the vinegar with an equivalent amount of freshly squeezed lemon juice and add 1 tablespoon (15 ml) of lemon zest.
- Greek dressing: add 1 teaspoon (4 ml) of dried oregano, dried basil and ground garlic.

78. "CHEESE" OF MACADAMIA AND CHIVES

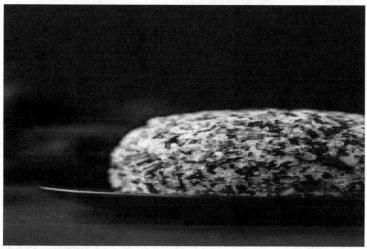

INGREDIENTS

- 2 cups (250 g) raw macadamia nuts
- 2 tablespoons (30 ml) freshly squeezed lemon juice
- teaspoon (1 ml) fine sea salt
- teaspoon (1 ml) black pepper
- teaspoon (1 ml) onion powder
- teaspoon (1 ml) ground garlic
- 1 or 2 tablespoons (15 to 30 ml) of hot water
- 3 or 4 tablespoons (45 to 60 ml) of fresh chives cut

PREPARATION

1. The "cheese" of nuts is a fantastic option for Keto diet enthusiasts who do not tolerate many dairy products but still love the delicious creaminess of the cheese. This recipe uses macadamia nuts, but other nuts can also be used. Cashews are very versatile, although they contain more carbohydrates (see the recipe for basic cashew cream. Always start with raw nuts, since roasted varieties usually contain unacceptable oils.

2. With a glass blender or a kitchen robot, beat the macadamia nuts with the lemon juice, salt, pepper, onion powder and ground garlic until it forms a thick paste and stumbles. Scratch the walls if necessary.

3. With the mixer or the kitchen robot running, add water little by little until the mixture acquires the desired consistency. It can be stopped when the "cheese" still has a light texture or continue beating until it is very homogeneous.

4. Pour the chives and press the switch several times to mix everything.

79. CARROT LEAF PESTO

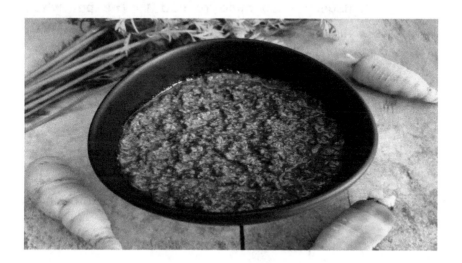

INGREDIENTS

- 1 cup (30 g) carrot leaves and stems
- cup (30 g) raw macadamia nuts
- cup (30 g) raw hazelnuts
- 1 crushed small garlic clove
- $\frac{1}{4}$ cup (25 g) grated Parmesan cheese
- cup (180 g) extra virgin olive oil Salt and pepper

PREPARATION

1. Carrot leaves are very underestimated. I usually keep mine to add to the pot when making a bone broth, but if I have enough broth I prepare a little of this pesto.
2. In a small kitchen robot, beat the carrot leaves, nuts, garlic and cheese until they mix well. Scratch the walls of the bowl.
3. With the kitchen robot running, gradually add the olive oil until the pesto acquires the desired consistency. Try and salt and pepper.

80. BUTTER WITH CHILLI PEPPER AND BACON

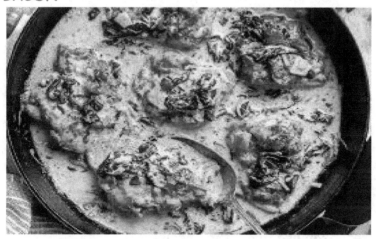

INGREDIENTS

- 2 slices of bacon (not too thick)
- cup (100 g) unsalted butter at room temperature 1 very thinly sliced garlic clove
- teaspoon (2 ml) sweet paprika
- teaspoon (2 ml) hot pepper
- teaspoon (2 ml) crushed dried oregano
- $\frac{1}{4}$ teaspoon (1 ml) ground cumin
- 1 / 8 teaspoon (0.5 ml) onion powder $\frac{1}{2}$ teaspoon (2 ml) kosher salt
- $\frac{1}{4}$ teaspoon (1 ml) black pepper

PREPARATION

1. Yes, you read that right; This recipe combines two of our favorite products, bacon and butter. It is perfect to melt on a juicy steak or a plate of scrambled eggs. For a change, try it with shrimp skewers, roasted Brussels sprouts or a very hot sweet potato the day you decide to take more carbohydrates.

2. Toast the bacon for about three minutes in a pan until it is crispy. Transfer it to a sheet of paper towels to drain it. Reserve bacon fat for use in another recipe.

3. Cut the butter into pieces and put them in a small bowl. Crush them with a fork.

4. Add garlic, sweet and spicy paprika, oregano, cumin, onion powder, salt and pepper, and mix well.

5. Crumble or chop the bacon. Add it to the butter and stir.

6. Spread the butter mixture on a piece of baking paper about 30 cm Shape cylinder and roll tightly. Twist the ends to close it.

7. Store the butter in the refrigerator until it is used (it can also be frozen).

81. CHICKEN LIVER PATE

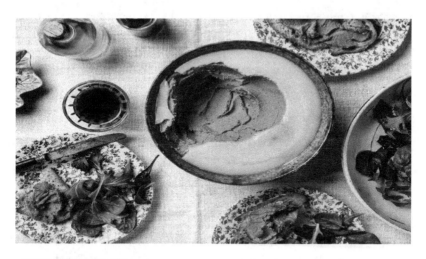

INGREDIENTS

- 225 g of chicken livers
- 6 tablespoons (85 g) of butter
- 2 tablespoons (30 ml) bacon fat
- small onion cut into rings 1 large clove garlic fillet
- 2 tablespoons (30 ml) red wine vinegar
- 1 tablespoon (15 ml) balsamic vinegar
- 1 teaspoon (5 ml) of Dijon mustard
- tablespoon (75 ml) of fresh cut rosemary Salt and pepper to taste
- Salt flakes (Maldon type) to decorate

PREPARATION

1. The liver is one of the healthiest foods that exist, so it is a pity that it has such a bad reputation. Hopefully this tasty pate will help you change your mind about this star food. It can be eaten with celery branches, cucumber slices or red peppers. And even with apple slices.

2. Remove the fibrous parts of the livers. Melt two tablespoons (30 ml) of the butter and bacon fat over medium heat in a medium skillet. Add the onion and livers and saute for six to eight minutes.

3. Pour the garlic and saute one more minute. Lower the heat a little and add the two types of vinegar, mustard and rosemary. Cook about five minutes, until almost all the liquid evaporates and the livers are well done.

4. Move the entire contents of the pan to a kitchen robot. Press the switch several times to mix everything. Scrape the walls of the bowl and add two tablespoons (30 g) of the butter. Process until you acquire one quite homogeneous texture. Scratch the bowl walls again. Add the other two tablespoons (30 g) of butter and process until it acquires a perfectly homogeneous texture.

5. Try and salt and pepper. Transfer the pasta to individual bowls and cover with transparent film. Store it in the fridge. Before serving, sprinkle each bowl with a little sea salt flake.

82. COCONUT BUTTER

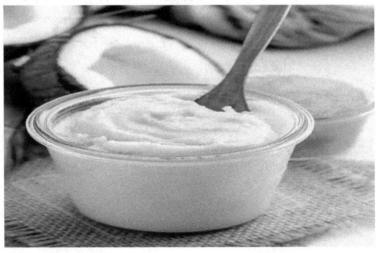

INGREDIENTS

- 4 cups (350 to 400 g) of unsweetened coconut flakes

PREPARATION

1. If you've never tried coconut butter, a pleasant surprise awaits you. You can add it to coffee or smoothies, mix it with root vegetables, use it in curried dishes or eat it spread in a thick layer on some apple slices or a piece of dark chocolate. In addition, it is the main ingredient of grease pumps. You will want to have a bottle always at hand!

2. If you use a kitchen robot: Put the coconut flakes in a kitchen robot and beat them for a maximum of fifteen minutes, scratching the walls if necessary (some kitchen robots take a little longer).
3. If you use a glass blender: Put half of the coconut flakes in the glass and beat for a minute. Add the rest and continue beating for a maximum of ten minutes, scratching the walls if necessary. Make sure the blender doesn't get too hot!
4. Transfer coconut butter to an airtight container until ready to use (it can be stored at room temperature). If necessary, heat it in the microwave for five to ten seconds before serving.
5. With both methods, coconut butter will go through three stages. First it will be very crumbled, then it will become a granulated liquid and, finally, it will acquire a homogeneous texture. If you are not sure that the process is complete, try it. The finished product should be homogeneous and slightly granulated, such as freshly ground nut butter.

83. SMOKED SALMON PATE

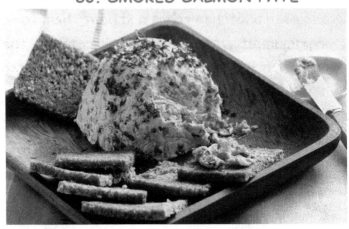

INGREDIENTS

- 4 tablespoons (60 g) of butter at room temperature
- 1 tablespoon (15 g) extra virgin olive oil
- 2 tablespoons (30 ml) chopped fresh chives
- 2 tablespoons (30 ml) of dried capers (30 ml)
- 2 tablespoons (30 ml) freshly squeezed lemon juice
- 225 g of cooked salmon fillet, without bones or skin
- 115 g smoked salmon cut into small cubes Salt and pepper to taste

PREPARATION

1. It is a fantastic way to take advantage of salmon leftovers. This preparation, full of healthy fats, can be taken at breakfast, lunch or dinner, or as a healthy snack. It is made in a matter of minutes, but it tastes so good that it is able to impress the diners of the most select dinner. Put a few tablespoons on some chicory or endive leaves to present it elegantly.

2. In a medium bowl, mix the butter and olive oil with a fork. Add the chives, capers and lemon juice.

3. Use a fork to divide the cooked salmon into small pieces and add it to the butter mixture. Add the smoked salmon and stir well, crushing it lightly. Fill a bowl, cover and store in the refrigerator until serving the pate.

84. OLIVE WITH NUTS

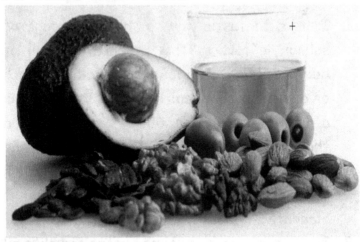

INGREDIENTS

- 1 cup (250 ml) of boneless olives (use a mixture of greens and blacks)
- 2 anchovy fillets in olive oil (see Tip)
- cup (60 ml) chopped walnuts 1 crushed garlic clove
- 1 tablespoon (15 ml) of drained capers
- 1 tablespoon (15 ml) chopped fresh basil
- 3 tablespoons (45 ml) extra virgin olive oil

PREPARATION

1. The traditional olive is a mixture of olives, capers, anchovies and onions crushed in the admiralty, and is usually served with small toasts. It is a fantastic way to introduce in our diet these little fish rich in omega fatty acids. The crunchy touch of nuts replaces that of toast. Serve this olive on slices of cucumber or red pepper, spread with it the baked chicken or add more olive oil to use as salad dressing.
2. In a small kitchen robot (or in a syrup), mix the ingredients and press the switch ten times. Scrape the walls of the bowl and continue pressing until the olive acquires the desired consistency.
3. Put in a bowl, cover with transparent film and put in the fridge until serving time.

85. SLOW COOKER CARNITAS

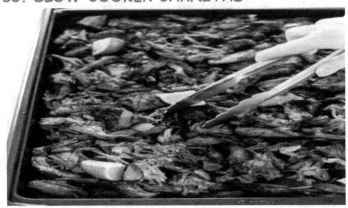

INGREDIENTS

- 1 teaspoon (5 ml) of kosher salt
- 1 teaspoon (5 ml) ground cumin
- 1 teaspoon (5 ml) dried oregano
- teaspoon (2 ml) black pepper 1 boneless pork shoulder (1.8 kg)
- 1 cup (250 ml) chicken or beef broth 1 orange thinly sliced
- Very chopped onion
- Fresh Cilantro Cut
- Diced Avocado
- Thinly sliced radishes
- Lime wedges
- Jalapeño Rings
- Lettuce or cabbage leaves

PREPARATION

1. If a busy week awaits me, on Sunday I prepare carnitas for the whole week. The best way to reheat them is to put them on the oven plate, under the grill.

2. In a small bowl, mix salt, cumin, oregano and pepper. Remove excess fat from meat (we are interested in keeping some fat, so only the large pieces will have to be removed). Rub the meat with the mixture of salt and spices.

3. Add the broth at the bottom of a slow cooker. Place the meat inside and cover with the orange slices. Cook it between eight and ten hours at low temperature (the preferred option) or six hours at high temperature.

4. Remove the meat carefully from the slow cooker and discard the orange slices. With two forks, shred the meat.

5. If desired, spread the shredded meat on a plate or baking dish. Turn on the grill at low temperature and place the oven rack about 10 cm from the heat. Place the meat dish under the grill and let it become crispy, making sure it does not burn.

6. Divide into portions and serve with optional ingredients. If desired, serve with lettuce or cabbage leaves to prepare some paleolithic tacos.

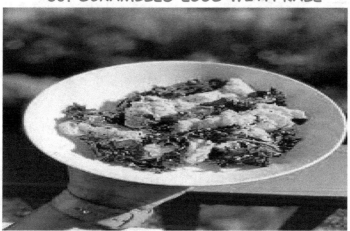

INGREDIENTS

- 2 tablespoons (30 ml) bacon fat or avocado oil
- cup (50 g) chopped red onion and 40 g chopped red pepper 1 clove garlic fillet
- 1 tablespoon (5 g) of sun-dried or baked tomatoes (see Note) 2 cups (475 g) of carnitas in slow cooker
- 1 teaspoon (5 ml) of kosher salt
- 1 teaspoon (5 ml) dried oregano
- $\frac{3}{4}$ teaspoon (4 ml) ground cumin Freshly ground black pepper
- 2 cups (30 g) of chopped kale leaves ($\frac{1}{2}$ bunch) $\frac{1}{2}$ lemon juice
- 1/3 cup (30 g) grated cheddar cheese

PREPARATION

1. This is a great way to take advantage of leftover carnitas to prepare another dish. I love having breakfast when I don't feel like eating eggs.
2. Heat the bacon fat in a large skillet over medium heat. Pour the onion and pepper. Fry for five minutes, until the vegetables begin to soften. Add the garlic and fry one more minute.
3. Incorporate tomatoes and meat. Mix until hot.
4. In a small bowl, mix the salt, oregano, cumin and pepper. Add to the pan and stir well.
5. Pour the chopped kale (it may have to be done twice, depending on the size of the pan). When the kale begins to soften, add the lemon juice and stir well.
6. Sprinkle with cheese evenly, reduce heat and cover.
7. Cook until the cheese is melted (if the pan is suitable for the oven, it can be placed under the grill to brown the top).
8. Divide into two portions and serve.

87. FAKE CUBAN SANDWICH

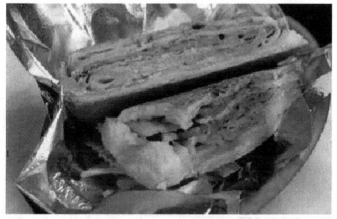

INGREDIENTS

- 1 teaspoon (5 ml) avocado oil
- 4 cups (1 kg) of carnitas in slow cooker
- 1 teaspoon (5 ml) of kosher salt
- Freshly ground black pepper
- $\frac{1}{2}$ lime juice
- 1 cup (250 ml) sliced pickles (normal or spicy, not sweet)
- 6 thin slices of cooked ham (of the best possible quality)
- 3 tablespoons (45 ml) of Dijon mustard
- 2 cups (180 g) shredded Swiss cheese

PREPARATION

1. Another fantastic idea to take advantage of leftover carnitas. This variant of the traditional Cuban sandwich eliminates the bread and leaves the best: the delicious filling. Eat it with a knife and fork or wrap it in cabbage leaves.

2. Place the oven rack at a distance between 10 and 15 cm from the grill and turn it on at the minimum temperature. Use avocado oil to grease the oven plate a little or a grill-ready dish. Spread the shredded pork forming a layer of about 2 cm. Season and sprinkle with lime juice. Place under the grill and gratin about two minutes, until the top begins to brown.

3. Remove the plate from the oven without turning off the grill. Arrange the cucumber slices, followed by the ham. Use the back of a spoon or spatula to carefully spread the mustard over the ham slices. Sprinkle the cheese in a homogeneous layer on top of the ham.

4. Put the plate back under the grill for one to two minutes to brown the part higher. Watch

the cheese so that it melts and begins to bubble and brown without burning.

88. MINCED MEAT OF THE CAVERNS WITH BUTTER ALMONDS

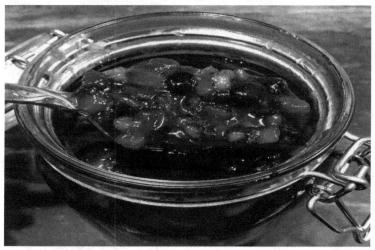

INGREDIENTS

- 700 g of minced beef
- 1 teaspoon (5 ml) Himalayan pink salt
- teaspoon (2 ml) ground pepper
- teaspoon (2 ml) ground cinnamon
- cup (120 ml) raw almond butter

PREPARATION

1. With such a simple recipe, the most important thing is the quality of the ingredients. I recommend wagyu minced meat, a type of Japanese cow similar to Kobe (if you can't find it in stores in your area, you can order it online). At first glance, this recipe may seem a bit odd, but try it the next time you need to resist for a long time. This dish will provide you with a lot of energy and a feeling of prolonged satiety that will allow you to take a six-hour walk through a rainforest. If it's your turn to cook, multiply the ingredients by five to feed your classmates.

2. In a medium skillet, brown the meat over medium heat for six to eight minutes until it is well done. Add salt, pepper and cinnamon. Stir well.

3. Add almond butter to tablespoons and stir vigorously. When well incorporated, remove from heat. Distribute in four bowls and serve immediately.

89. LIGHT TUNA BRAISED WITH HERB AND LIME DRESSING

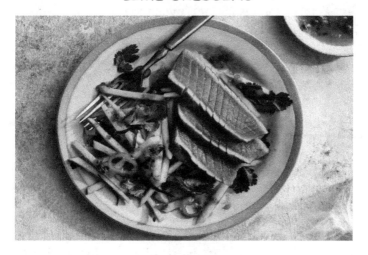

INGREDIENTS

- 170 g of light tuna steak for sushi
- Sea salt
- Freshly ground black pepper
- 2 tablespoons (30 ml) avocado oil

Herbs + Lima Dress

- 1 cup (150 g) fresh cilantro
- 1 cup (150 g) fresh parsley
- 1 teaspoon (5 ml) lime zest
- The juice of 2 small limes (1½ to 2 tablespoons; 25 ml)
- 2 tablespoons (30 ml) tamari (gluten-free soy sauce)
- 1 tablespoon (15 ml) roasted sesame oil
- 1 clove garlic, thinly sliced or crushed
- A 2.5 cm piece of fresh ginger, finely sliced or grated
- ½ cup (60 to 120 ml) of extra virgin olive oil or avocado oil A pinch of red pepper in small pieces (optional)

PREPARATION

1. Preparing light seared tuna may seem difficult, but it is not. If you want a quick and simple dish

that impresses your guests, this is ideal. Serve the tuna with a simple green salad.

2. Cut the tuna steak into two or three elongated rectangular portions. Pepper the two sides of each piece.

3. Put the cilantro and parsley in a small kitchen robot (see Note). Chop the herbs. Add the zest and lime juice, tamari, sesame oil, garlic and ginger. Press the switch several times to mix well. Scratch the walls of the bowl.

4. With the robot running, slowly add the olive oil. Scratch the walls again and press the switch several times. If the sauce is too thick, add more oil until the desired consistency is obtained.

5. In a large skillet, heat the avocado oil over medium-high heat until it is quite hot. Gently place the tuna in the oil and braise for one minute on each side without moving. The tuna will be pink in the center. If you want to do more, you will have to extend the cooking time a bit.

6. Remove the tuna from the pan, cut it into pieces about 15 mm thick, add the dressing and serve.

90. FILLED TOMATOES

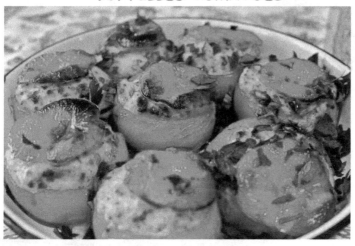

INGREDIENTS

- 6 medium tomatoes
- 225 g minced beef
- 1 teaspoon (5 ml) dried basil
- ½ teaspoon (2 ml) of kosher salt
- teaspoon (1 ml) black pepper 6 medium eggs

PREPARATION

1. This simple recipe is better if it is prepared with tomatoes fresh from the garden. If you prefer, you can use turkey or chicken, and even lamb.
2. Preheat the oven to 200 ° C. With a sharp knife, cut the stems of the tomatoes. Carefully remove the seeds with a spoon and discard them.
3. Put the tomatoes in a small pan suitable for the oven or use a plate for large cavity muffins. Bake five minutes.
4. Brown the meat in a medium skillet about twenty-five minutes, until it is well done. Season with salt and pepper and add basil.
5. Remove the tomatoes from the oven and turn on the grill only (if adjustable, at low temperature). Divide the meat into six portions and place it in the tomatoes with a spoon.
6. Shell an egg inside each tomato and salt and pepper a little more.
7. Put the tomatoes in the oven for about five minutes, at a distance of 10 to 15 cm from the grill, until the egg whites are curdled and the yolks still liquid.

91. THE BEST ROAST CHICKEN

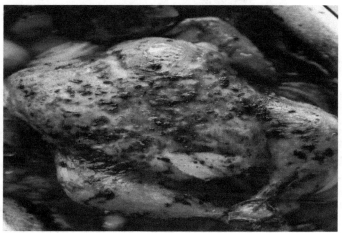

INGREDIENTS

- 4 half boneless and skinless chicken breasts (approximately 1 kg)
- 3 tablespoons (45 ml) kosher salt
- Ice cubes
- 2 tablespoons (30 ml) avocado oil
- 2 tablespoons (30 ml) of chicken seasoning (make sure it doesn't have any added sugar)

PREPARATION

1. Surely this tasty chicken will quickly become one of the family's favorite dishes. It is delicious accompanied by a varied salad, wrapped in cabbage leaves with a portion of Primal mayonnaise or simply served with your favorite roasted vegetables. The secret is brine, which leaves the chicken tasty and tender.

2. Cut each chicken breast diagonally into three elongated portions.

3. Bring a cup (240 ml) of water to a boil. Mix the boiling water and salt in a large metal or glass bowl. When the salt dissolves, pour a liter of cold water and some ice cubes. Add the chicken pieces and cover them with 2-5 cm of cold water. Put in the fridge fifteen minutes.

4. Drain the chicken. If you want to avoid being salty, rinse it now, although it is not necessary. Mix the oil and the chicken seasoning in the empty bowl. Then put the chicken in the oil. Let stand for a few minutes.

5. Heat a grill over medium-high heat. When hot, place the chicken pieces and cover. Roast for about four minutes, turn around and continue roasting for three or four more minutes, until the internal temperature reaches 75 ° C.
6. Remove the chicken from the grill and serve.

92. CHICKEN SKEWERS

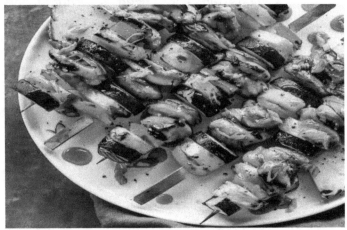

INGREDIENTS

- 1 kg half boneless and skinless chicken breasts
- 24 small mushrooms (approximately 225 g)
- 1 large yellow onion
- 2 peppers (the color you prefer)
- cup (60 ml) avocado oil 1 teaspoon (5 ml) dried oregano
- 1 teaspoon (5 ml) dried basil $\frac{1}{2}$ teaspoon (2 ml) ground garlic $\frac{1}{2}$ teaspoon (2 ml) kosher salt
- $\frac{1}{2}$ teaspoon (2 ml) black pepper
- 8 short skewers (soaked in water if they are made of wood or bamboo)

PREPARATION

1. Skewers are my favorite dish when people come home to enjoy an informal summer barbecue. You can prepare them in advance, or even let the guests prepare them. As they roast in a moment, you won't have to take care of the grill while your guests have fun.

2. Cut each chicken breast into eight or ten pieces of similar size and put them in a glass bowl. Wash the mushrooms and remove their feet. Cut the onion and peppers into large pieces. Put everything in another bowl.

3. Mix the oil and seasonings. Pour half of the mixture into each bowl and stir well. Put the two bowls in the fridge and marinate for twenty minutes.

4. Mount the skewers alternating chicken and vegetables on skewers. Preheat the iron to medium-high temperature.

5. Put the skewers on the grill (or under the grill) for about three minutes on each side, turning them so that they brown well everywhere, about

6. Ten or twelve minutes in total. Check the chicken with an instant read thermometer to

make sure it is well done (the internal temperature should be 75 ° C).

7. Move the skewers to a source and serve.

93. SHRIMP AND ASPARAGUS TRAY

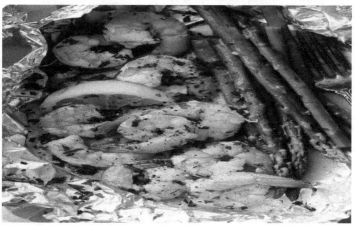

INGREDIENTS

- 2 tablespoons (30 ml) avocado oil
- 3 sliced garlic cloves
- 4 tablespoons (60 g) of butter
- 1 bunch of asparagus (450 g)
- 2 teaspoons (10 ml) of kosher salt
- 1 teaspoon (5 ml) freshly ground black pepper
- 680 g peeled shrimp
- ½ teaspoon (1-2 ml) of chopped red pepper (optional) 1 medium lemon cut in half
- 1 cup (90 g) shredded Parmesan cheese
- 2 tablespoons (30 ml) chopped fresh parsley (optional)

PREPARATION

1. I don't like to wash casseroles at all, so my thing is to prepare food in a single container. In

addition, this simple dish is made in less than twenty minutes. You'll love it!

2. Preheat the oven to 200 ° C. In a small skillet, heat the avocado oil over medium heat. Sauté the garlic until they release their aroma and without getting brown, about three minutes. Add the butter and cook until it begins to bubble. Remove from the fire.

3. Remove the hard ends of the asparagus and put the tips on the oven plate. Pour over two tablespoons (30 ml) of the butter with garlic and give them a few turns to cover them well. Spread them in a single layer and sprinkle them with half the salt and pepper. Put them in the oven for five minutes, until they are tender and lightly toasted.

4. Place the asparagus in one half of the plate. Put the prawns in the other half. Pour over the rest of the butter with garlic and give them some turns to cover them well. Spread them in a single layer and sprinkle them with the rest of the salt and pepper. Add the red pepper, if used. Squeeze the lemon over the prawns and cut it into quarters. Put the rooms between the prawns.

5. Sprinkle the Parmesan cheese only on the asparagus and put the plate in the oven for five to eight minutes, until the prawns are opaque. Pour the parsley over the prawns, if used, and serve immediately.

94. SAUSAGES WITH KALE

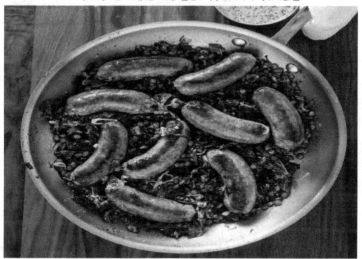

INGREDIENTS

- 1 bunch of kale of any variety
- $\frac{1}{2}$ diced medium onion
- 1 package of chicken sausages
- 2 tablespoons (30 ml) coconut oil or avocado
- 2 tablespoons (30 ml) of butter
- 8 clean and sliced mushrooms
- 1 teaspoon (5 ml) of kosher salt
- $\frac{1}{2}$ teaspoon (2 ml) black pepper
- 1 cup (250 ml) chicken broth (preferably homemade)
- $\frac{1}{4}$ teaspoon (1 ml) chopped red pepper (optional)

PREPARATION

1. If any of your friends or family members say they don't like kale, give them a taste of this dish. This recipe can be customized to taste, adding the desired vegetables and any type of sausage. Try different combinations to see which one you like best. However, be sure to choose sausages that only contain clean ingredients, without added sugars, nitrates and so on.

2. With a sharp knife, cut the thick stalks of the kale present in the leaf portions. Chop them into pieces of a size similar to diced onion. Cut the kale leaves into thin strips.

3. Cut the sausages into 2.5 cm pieces. Heat a tablespoon (15 ml) of oil in a large pan. Put half of the sausages in a single layer and fry until golden brown. Turn them over and fry them two minutes on the other side. Remove them and repeat the operation with the other half of the sausages. Remove them from the pan.

4. Heat the other tablespoon (15 ml) of oil in medium heat on it pan. Add the onion and cut kale stalks and fry the vegetables for about five minutes, until they begin to soften. Push the vegetables to the edge of the pan and melt the butter in the center. Add the mushrooms and sauté them for a few minutes. Add salt and pepper. Stir well.

5. Add the kale leaves and mix everything. Fry for three to five minutes, until the leaves are soft. Return the sausages to the pan along with the

broth and chopped red pepper, if used. Raise the fire a little. When the liquid begins to boil, lower the heat and wait for almost everything to evaporate. Try and add salt if necessary. Serve right away.

95. BAKED SALMON WITH DILL AIOLI

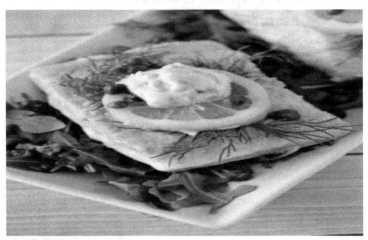

INGREDIENTS

- 4 salmon fillets with skin, approximately 170 g each
- tablespoon (7.5 ml) avocado oil Zest of ½ large lemon
- Kosher salt
- Freshly ground black pepper

Alioli To Drop

- ½ cup (120 ml) of Primal Kitchen mayonnaise or other mayonnaise suitable for the paleolithic diet
- 2 small sliced garlic cloves
- 2 teaspoons (15 ml) freshly squeezed lemon juice
- 1 tablespoon (15 ml) chopped fresh dill

- teaspoon (1 ml) kosher salt
- teaspoon (1 ml) freshly ground black pepper
  zest of $\frac{1}{2}$ large lemon

PREPARATION

1. This salmon fillet baked at low temperature melts in the mouth. Prepared like this, the salmon is pretty pink, so don't be alarmed when you take it out of the oven and it still looks raw. On the contrary, it will be the best made fish you've ever eaten!

2. Preheat the oven to 135 ° C. Put the salmon fillets in an iron pot or baking dish. Mix the oil with half the lemon zest and paint the top of the fish. Salt and pepper Bake the salmon between sixteen and eighteen minutes, until it can be divided into small pieces with a fork.

3. While the salmon is in the oven, mix the mayonnaise with the garlic, zest and lemon juice, dill, salt and pepper.

4. Serve the salmon accompanied by the aioli.

96. TURKEY AND CABBAGE ROLLS

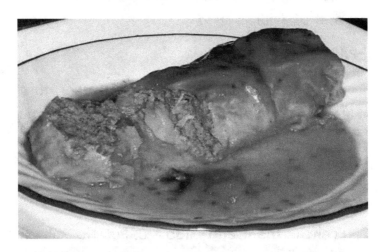

INGREDIENTS

- 2 cabbage leaves, the bigger the better
- 4 slices of good quality turkey breast (no added sugar or nitrites or other harmful ingredients)
- 4 slices of bacon passed through the pan
- 2 slices of Swiss cheese cut in half
- ½ cup (120 ml) paleolithic coleslaw

PREPARATION

1. After experimenting with different options, I have concluded that cabbage is the ingredient that best substitutes flatbread and Mexican tortillas. It has a very mild flavor, and its large and thick leaves hold the filling very well. This sandwich is a bit complicated to eat, but it is great.

2. With a sharp knife, remove the thick central stem of the cabbage (you may have to cut the leaf a little, leaving it in the shape of a heart).

3. In the center of each leaf, layer two slices of turkey, two slices of bacon and two half slices of cheese, leaving a margin on the edges. With a spoon, put $\frac{1}{4}$ cup (60 ml) of coleslaw on each leaf, near the top (away from the end of the stem).

4. Starting at the top, wrap the coleslaw with the tip of the leaf and roll up the sandwich. Tuck the edges like a burrito. Close the rolls with two chopsticks each and cut in half to serve.

97. CRISPY TUNA SALAD

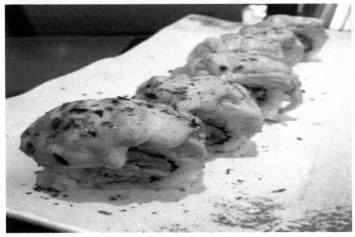

INGREDIENTS

- 2 tuna cans of 140 g each (do not drain)
- $\frac{1}{2}$ cup (120 ml) of Primal Kitchen mayonnaise or other mayonnaise suitable for the paleolithic diet
- 2 tablespoons (30 ml) drained capers
- 1 diced celery stalk
- 1 small carrot, diced
- 4 diced radishes
- Salt and pepper to taste
- cup (60 g) filleted almonds 2 tablespoons (15 g) sunflower seeds

PREPARATION

1. Another idea to use cabbage leaves. You can also enjoy this salad with vegetables, with slices of radish, with cucumber chips or alone. Be sure to select tuna caught sustainably and packed in water or olive oil.
2. Empty the tuna in a bowl together with the canning liquid. Crumble it with a fork. Add the mayonnaise, capers, celery, carrots and radishes. Try and salt and pepper.
3. Chop the almonds with a chef's knife. Just before serving, add them to the tuna salad and sprinkle everything with sunflower seeds.

98. Chicken Stuffed With Nopales

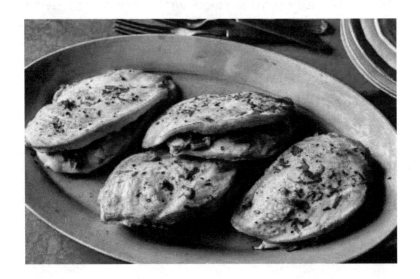

INGREDIENTS

- 1 tablespoon of oil
- 1/2 cups white onion, filleted
- 1 cup of nopal, cut into strips and cooked
- enough of salt
- enough of oregano
- enough of pepper
- 4 chicken breasts, flattened
- 1 cup of Oaxaca cheese, shredded
- 1 tablespoon of oil, for sauce
- 3 cloves of garlic, chopped, for sauce
- 1 white onion, cut in eighths, for sauce
- 6 tomatoes, cut into quarters, for sauce582

- 1/4 cups of fresh coriander, fresh, for sauce
- 4 guajillo chilies, for the sauce
- 1 tablespoon of allspice, for sauce
- 1 Cup of chicken broth, for sauce
- 1 pinch of salt, for sauce

PREPARATION

6. For the filling, heat a pan over medium heat with the oil, cook the onion with the nopales until they stop releasing drool, season to your liking with salt, pepper and oregano. Reservation.

7. On a board, place the chicken breasts, stuffed with the nopales and Oaxaca cheese, roll up, season with salt, pepper and a little oregano. If necessary secure with a toothpick.

8. Heat a grill over high heat and cook the chicken rolls until they are cooked through. Cut the rolls and reserve hot.

9. For the sauce, heat a pan over medium heat with the oil, cook the garlic with the onion until you get a golden color, add the tomato, the coriander, the guajillo chili, the allspice, the coriander seeds. Cook for 10 minutes, fill

with the chicken broth, season with salt, and continue cooking for 10 more minutes. Chill slightly.

10. Blend the sauce until you get a homogeneous mixture. Serve on a plate as a mirror, place the chicken on top and enjoy.

99. Mini Meatloaf With Bacon

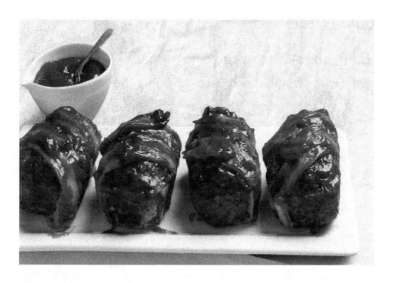

INGREDIENTS

- 1 kilo of ground beef
- 1/2 cups of ground bread
- 1 egg
- 1 cup onion, finely chopped
- 2 tablespoons garlic, finely minced
- 4 tablespoons ketchup
- 1 tablespoon mustard
- 2 teaspoons parsley, finely chopped
- enough of salt
- enough of pepper
- 12 slices of bacon
- enough of ketchup sauce, to varnish
- enough of parsley, to decorate

PREPARATION

6. Preheat the oven to 180 ° C.
7. In a bowl, mix the ground beef with the breadcrumbs, the egg, the onion, the garlic, the ketchup, the mustard, the parsley, the salt and the pepper.
8. Take approximately 150 g of the meat mixture and shape it in a circular shape with the help of your hands. Wrap with bacon and place on a greased cookie sheet or waxed paper. Brush the top of the cupcakes and bacon with ketchup.
9. Bake for 15 minutes or until the meat is cooked and the bacon is golden brown.
10. Serve with parsley, accompanied by salad and pasta.

100. Chicken Wire With Cheese

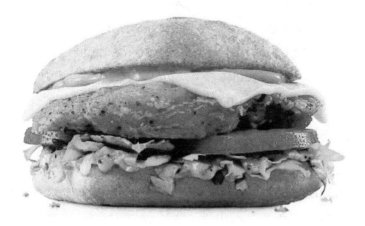

INGREDIENTS

- 1/2 cups chorizo, crumbled
- 1/2 cups bacon, chopped
- 2 tablespoons garlic, finely minced
- 1 red onion, cut into chunks
- 2 chicken breasts, skinless, boneless, diced
- 1 cup mushroom, filleted
- 1 yellow bell pepper, cut into chunks

- 1 red bell pepper, cut into chunks
- 1 bell pepper, orange cut into chunks
- 1 pumpkin, cut into half moons
- 1 pinch of salt and pepper
- 1 cup of Manchego cheese, grated
- to taste of corn tortillas, to accompany
- to taste of sauce, to accompany
- to taste of lemon, to accompany

PREPARATION

4. Heat a skillet over medium heat and fry the chorizo and bacon until golden brown. Add the garlic and onion and cook until transparent. Add the chicken, season with salt and pepper and cook until golden brown.

5. Once the chicken is cooked, add the vegetables one at a time, cooking for a few minutes before adding the next. Finally, add the cheese and cook 5 more minutes so that it melts, rectify the seasoning.

6. Serve the wire very hot accompanied by corn tortillas, salsa and lemon.

CONCLUSION

Low-fat diets are considered a popular method of weight loss.

However, low-carb diets are linked to greater short-term weight loss, along with increased fat loss, reduced hunger, and better blood sugar control.

While more studies are needed on the long-term effects of each diet, studies show that low-carbohydrate diets can be just as effective for weight loss as low-fat diets – and can offer several additional benefits to weight loss. health.

Whether you choose a low-carb or low-fat diet, keep in mind that maintaining a long-term eating pattern is one of the most critical factors for success in both weight loss and overall health.

CPSIA information can be obtained
at www.ICGtesting.com
Printed in the USA
LVHW080546110322
713213LV00002B/19